For our sons
Philipp, Florian, and Christopher-Ray Jr.
Knowledge has no final aspect!

FAKTuell-Verlag
We make it easy!

We would like to thank all physicians practicing the New Medicine who contributed with their commitment to the realization of this book.
Special thanks go to Dr. Ryke Geerd Hamer,
who was even willing to go to prison for his patients.

FAKTuell-Verlag
We make it easy!

factor-L
Handbook of the New Medicine
The Truth about Dr. Hamer's Discoveries
Conflicts – Triggers – Courses
regarding cancer and other curable diseases

Authors:
Monika Berger-Lenz
Christopher Ray

The New Medicine in practice:
Andreas Kroitzsch

Specialized Book © 2005
FAKTuell-Verlag

Editor
Christopher Ray

The legend
The omnipotence of the so-called traditional medicine is faltering, the patients become responsible. Alternatives are in demand. The New Medicine of the German physician, Dr. Ryke Geerd Hamer, offers this alternative. It is clear, easy to understand, and, in 2003, was confirmed to be scientific by the expert opinion of Professor Dr. Hans-Ulrich Niemitz.

The book
The second factor-L volume about the New Medicine according to Dr. Hamer offers deeper insight in the processes of so-called diseases. It addresses the triggers of a conflict (DHS), which, in terms of the traditional medicine, is called disease, as well as the courses of so-called diseases Dr. Ryke Geerd Hamer recognized and classified as Meaningful Special Biological Programs (SBS).

Note:
This book is not a medical guidebook. It can, however, help you with the decision to take more responsibility for yourself and your health. With more knowledge about Dr. Hamer's New Medicine, you are in charge again of designing your life. Diseases and diagnoses become less scary.

The authors:
For years, Monika Berger-Lenz and Christopher Ray have been making a name for themselves as journalists and authors of specialized books by conducting intensive background research and presenting the results in a generally understandable way. Together, they operate Germany's oldest online newspaper, FAKTuell.de (since 1982).

Verlag
FAKTuell ® Redaktion und Verlag
Berger-Lenz
An den Birken 5
D-02827 Görlitz
Germany

Cover & Layout: Claudia von Hausen * GOpress.de
English Translation by Carola Kern * carolakern.com

Production: Book on Demand GmbH
Retail bookseller:
BoD/LIBRI (D) * Ingram, Baker & Taylor (USA) * Bertrams and Gardners (UK)

ISBN: 978-3-9809203-6-0
(2006: ISBN: 3-9809203-6-4)
EAN: 9783980920399
Price: 24,80 €

FAKTuell ® is a registered trademark of the FAKTuell editorial department Berger-Lenz

factor-L
Handbook of the New Medicine
The Truth about Dr. Hamer's Discoveries
Conflicts – Triggers – Courses
regarding cancer and other curable diseases

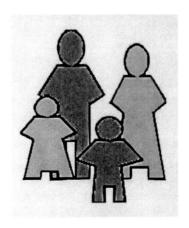

Hamer Focus = HH
(original: Hamerscher Herd)
Hamer Foci = HH
(original: Hamersche Herde)
Dirk Hamer Syndrome = DHS
(original: Dirk-Hamer-Syndrom)
Meaningful Special Biological Program = SBS
(original: Sinnvolles Biologisches Sonderprogramm)

Original:
faktor-L
Handbuch Neue Medizin
Die Wahrheit über Dr. Hamers Entdeckung
Konflikte - Auslöser - Verlauf
bei Krebs und anderen heilbaren Krankheiten
ISBN: 3-9809203-8-0
EAN: 9783980920384

Prologue

- Notification
- Belief Knowledge
- Dr. Hamer's New Medicine
- The formula: DHS – HH – SBS

More than 30 years ago, I entitled an article about Frank Stelzer and his free piston engine *"An inventor is a goofball"*. Someone or other who, at that time, read this 30-point headline probably may have thought that it wasn't the best way to begin a friendship. Frank Stelzer read the rest of the article, called me and said, *"That's right, but...."* *"But what?"* I asked. *"Unless the invention speaks,"* he responded. Then he invited me, demonstrated the Stelzer engine, and made the invention speak.

Tip:
If you never liked prologues, or you would like to go straight to the topic Conflicts and the New Medicine, turn directly to Introduction to the New Medicine by Andreas Kroll/sch on page 15!
The editor

Since that time we have been friends. Very good friends! And Stelzer turned "his" introductory sentence into a trademark: *"An inventor is a goofball – unless the invention speaks!"*

I am telling you about this, for, regarding Dr. Hamer's New Medicine we are dealing with a similar phenomenon. Like Stelzer, who turned everything that was imaginable in engine manufacturing upside down, and only received buying offers intended to keep his invention in the drawer, because his engine practically runs without wear, Dr. Ryke Geerd Hamer, with the new Medicine, has also turned everything upside down in his area.
And: "The invention speaks!"

If you know our throwaway society, which turned sales into a god and consumption into his apostles, you won't be surprised that Hamer hasn't found a lobby either among those who have the power and the money. On the contrary. Someone like Geerd Hamer jeopardizes the income and the position of power of the ruling people, which was the main reason why he was arrested in France in the fall of 2004. Seventy-year-old Dr. Hamer is supposed to serve three years in prison. But that is another story, which would go beyond the scope of this book. If you would like to know more about the personal history of Dr. Hamer, you are be best served by reading his autobiography *Einer gegen alle*. Even if you don't agree with all of his conclusions and assumptions regarding his persecution, they are worth knowing about. Everyone can then form his or her own opinion accordingly.

It is easier when it comes to the discovery of the New Medicine, where Hamer didn't leave any room for speculation. There is no room for belief or personality cult; there is only this one way of comprehension that, ultimately, gives us the certainty to be among the knowing. As is the case with any other education based on assured knowledge, the application of the New Medicine always leaves a result that can be checked. The scientific basis we often miss painfully - in the truest sense of the meaning - in the traditional medicine constitutes the foundation of Dr. Hamer's discovery.

Hamer himself never left any room for exceptions. His statement is clear and precise without any room for speculation: "If there is only one single case the New Medicine can't be applied to, it is wrong!" The New Medicine proves itself again and again with every single case. The formula: DHS – HH – SBS, which will be explained at length in this book, doesn't allow for exceptions. The New Medicine knows no "maybe", no "possibly", and no "potentially." Hamer's discovery puts the key to the so-called diseases in our hands. The knowledge of the principles of the New Medicine helps us lose the fear of the diseases, because we understand the biological processes and can predict them in their entirety.

But it is the small checkable truths we speak every day and have internalized since childhood in such a way that often prevents us from taking one more step towards understanding. Every one of us has been in a situation that was "hard to stomach" or "got under his or her skin?" These are all discreet clues showing that we carry the mechanisms and principles of the New Medicine in our sub-conscience. They are wasted – as long as we are not familiar with Hamer's New Medicine. It's like learning the times tables. Not until we know that two is the sum (result) of one plus one can we find our way to mathematics via digits and work with them sensibly. Knowledge always provides us with added value. This book helps you generate added value from your latent knowledge of the connection between situations and conditions.
You should be willing to leave well-trodden paths. The ability to change the point of view in order to get to know new perspectives will also be helpful. You get the chance to replace old fears with new knowledge. Needless to say, that comes with a price tag. You will have to take personal responsibility if you want to benefit from your new knowledge. The opinion of your environment, especially that of traditional physicians, politicians, and the pharmaceutical industry is contradictory to your newly acquired knowledge.

That is inconvenient, because you are inconvenient for the prevailing opinion. Particularly, if you realize for yourself that knowledge and belief are complete opposites. In the past, you have given away your trust concerning medicine and health and you believed in the traditional physicians. You believed that they'd know. This belief is the price you pay for your new knowledge of Hamer's New Medicine. There are no gods in white coats. And – and that is important – the New Medicine won't provide any substitute gods for you, not even one. The discoverer of the New Medicine, Dr. Ryke Geerd Hamer, can't take the orphaned throne either. He is a discoverer, not an inventor or even a savior. Even if some of his supporters would like to press him in that position in order to push the responsibility towards him.

If you want to give the responsibility for yourself to Dr. Hamer or somebody else, you have not understood the New Medicine, which requires knowledge and makes belief (ignorance!) redundant. You can't believe in science, you can just practice and understand it. All you need to do so is common sense. An excellent education based on "memorizing" isn't necessary, especially not with Dr. Hamer's New Medicine. Natural laws are so plausible that everybody can check them by watching his or her own body; even if he or she was an illiterate person who would be introduced to the New Medicine by a reader or taleteller, because we all know our body and many of the so-called diseases. We are all experienced and competent specialists in this area.

With the assistance of a handbook that explains the New Medicine, we can find the causes of our so-called diseases ourselves and lead the ongoing processes to what the traditional medicine calls healing. The processes that really take place are Meaningful Special Biological Programs (SBS). And these are the processes Hamer discovered, catalogued, and described in simple words in order to give the control over our body back to us again.

If you are not sure whether you have the right to think for yourself and question the traditional medicine, for your legitimation, I would like to quote an impressive sentence by the Swiss theologian, Kurt Marti:

> *Where would we be if we all just said*
> *"...where would we be" – and nobody would go*
> *to see where we would be if we went.*
> *—Kurt Marti*

Much too often we are kept from new findings and further personal development by being told that certain things have always been done a certain way. Or, it isn't our place to question because somebody studied something and, therefore, knows better and can do it better than us laymen can. And we yield to these alleged arguments only too willingly. It isn't right nor is it true, but, of course, it is always convenient. It is a familiar excuse for not having to think and take responsibility for yourself.

Theodore Sturgeon, an exceptionally gifted writer, put the demand on us in his own words, also hitting the nail on the head. Here is an excerpt from an interview:

Ask the Next Question!
An interview with Theodore Sturgeon
Interviewed by Dave Duncan

Could you explain the significance of your personal trademark, which is the letter Q with an arrow through the middle, pointing to the right?

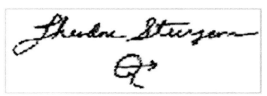

It means, "Ask the next question." Ask the next question, and the next, and the one that follows. It's the symbol of everything humanity has ever created, and it is the reason it has been created. This guy is sitting in a cave, saying, "Why can't man fly?" Well, that's the question. The answer may not help him, but the question has been asked.

The next question is what? How? And that's how people all through the ages have been trying to find the answer to that question. We've found the answer and we do fly. This is true of every accomplishment, whether it's technology or literature, poetry, political systems or anything else. That is it. Ask the next question. And the one after that.
Source: © Dave Duncan

This short interlude is supposed to show that it is legitimate for us to question everything the moment we change from the niche of belief to the broad field of knowledge. Curiosity is the best guidepost. If we don't push ourselves, we have to accept that others do it for us.

We learned the saying that smart people give in just to find out that the ignorant people lead the world if we stick to this "wisdom". If we have internalized that, we are ready to take the liberty of having a different view on things. We find that our perspectives are a result of our point of view, not only in geography, but also in all life situations.

Only if we are willing to check our point of view and give up the position we are currently adopting are we gaining a new view on things. You can only check points of view if you are willing to leave them for the check. Only if you leave (or question) your point of view will you be able to check it. That doesn't necessarily mean that you have to give it up for good.

If the view across the fence doesn't open any better perspectives, we can always go back again to our point of view. We will find that our point of view is now stronger, more confident. And our perspective has gained sharpness.

Every time we check our point of view we increase our situation. We create a safer foundation for ourselves; one that we have successfully checked to see whether it is flawed. If we change our point of view for good reasons, the new one is always safer than the old one - until we realize that another check is necessary. We should always leave this option open because we have to remain flexible (!!!) in order to find our footing. There are no final "truths".

Knowledge is always a snapshot of an ongoing process. That's why we have to check our positions again and again, so that we are not among the backward people who cling to antiquated points of view; the Labelers, as Sturgeon calls them. We have the freedom to learn from experience, including the experience of others. This book is dedicated to that freedom.

We can, may, and have to remind ourselves over and over again that the world isn't static. Knowledge is something that wants to be acquired, and develops its quality only if we use, check, and question it and constantly extend it. In order for us to become aware of that again, I chose the introduction from a volume of short stories by Theodore Sturgeon where he describes these mechanisms very impressively.

Note:
In the early 70s, Isaac Asimov, Walter Ernsting (Clark Darlton), Ted Sturgeon, and me exchanged letters, in which we talked about the prejudices (not only) against science fiction and the preference for stereotyped philosophies.
At that time, Ted Sturgeon sent us his introduction for a SF volume, in which he dealt with that particular topic in his matchless Art final.
In memory of Ted, who hit the nail right on the head, I pass that text on to you. Do something with it!
Christopher Ray

A Word in Advance
By Theodore Sturgeon

"So, now you also write pornography?" These words were recently expressed by a friend of Philip José Farmer. The question seems simple and honest. Obviously, it was asked by a human being who had the sincere feeling that he can define his own words and probably acted on the assumption that the terms he used were self-explanatory to a degree that they didn't need any definition.

There are a huge number of honest and well-meaning people who can, without hesitation, define:

Theodore Sturgeon,
Pornography,
God,
Right,
Evil,
Human rights,
Law and Order,
Science fiction,
Communism,
Freedom,
Honourable peace,
Obscenity,
Love,

and think, act, and legislate, and sometimes burn, imprison, and kill on the basis of their definitions. These are the Labelers, and they are without exception the most lethal and destructive force any species has ever faced on this or any other planet.

I will explain to you in a clear and simple way why:
One rarely comes across simple truths. Actually, everything that looks like the truth is subject to questions and modifications.
"Water always flows uphill."
At what temperature? And where – for example in an Apollo capsule or at a siphon spout?
"Only girls wear skirts."
Would you like to take on a battalion of the kilt-wearing Black Watch or a company of the rock-hard Greek Evzones? (They even wear skirts with laces!)
"E=MC^2", said Albert Einstein, the shining god of relativism, *"but it could also be a local phenomenon."*

The lethal destructiveness attached to the labeling is the fact that labelers, without exception, ignore the most fundamental basis of all characteristics of the entire universe – transformation: that is, the flowing and the change. If he stops and reflects (which, sure enough, is not a habit of his), the labeler has to admit that even rocks and mountains change, that planets and the stars change, and that they haven't stop changing due to the purely local and tiny detail that he accidentally labeled them at some point.

Transformation is more obvious in what we call life than in any other area. It is not enough to say that living things change; one has to go further and also say that life is change. Things that don't change act in opposition to the laws of the universe; things that don't change aren't alive, and life can't exist in the presence of things that don't change.

For that reason the labeler is lethal.
He is of damaging influence. His order is always, Stop! He is the friend of death and the enemy of life. He doesn't want to endure things as they really are; he can't endure them...moving, flowing, changing; he wants them to last.

Why?
I assume because of a very normal longing for safety. He wants to feel safe. He doesn't know that he mistakes stasis for stability. If only everything would stop, if the Today and the Tomorrow could just be like yesterday (for, he doesn't look at the Yesterday carefully enough, so he believes that yesterday everything was motionless, peaceful, and law-abiding – which, of course, it wasn't), he could really feel safe.

He doesn't understand that in the protective church of his choice he can meet respectable older women in clothes that used to be forbidden (older believers will remember that) not only on the street but also at the beach.

He has forgotten that, not so long ago, our species was overcome by something similar to a culture shock, because Clark Gable in his role as Rhett Butler used the word "*Damn*".

He conveniently ignores all evidence, all truths, and he labels instead. He is absolutely lethal, so keep your eyes open if you meet him.
© Theodore Sturgeon

While we are writing this book, the discoverer of the New Medicine is in a prison in France; he has been there for more than a year now. Labelers locked Dr. Hamer up there. What they couldn't lock up is his discovery. For, the truth can't be locked up.

Isolated in his cell, Dr. Hamer is troubled by fears that people could falsify his discovery and defame him. The authors of this book aren't immune to suspicions either. Therefore, we assured ourselves of the cooperation of a generally accepted expert who, more than 15 years ago, was taught Hamer's New Medicine by Dr. Hamer himself.

Andreas Kroitzsch belongs to the relatively small circle of experienced practitioners of the New Medicine. We are happy that Andreas Kroitzsch, by providing his introduction to the New Medicine, helped us turn this book into a comprehensible standard work of Hamer's New Medicine.

We all learn best from experience. Other experts of the New Medicine contributed their experience as well to make the practical processes transparent for all those involved. This book documents the triggers of all so-called diseases, which Hamer calls conflicts, using many comprehensible examples. Now it is your turn to check your points of view and gain new perspectives.

Görlitz, October 25, 2005
Monika Berger-Lenz
Christopher Ray

The Turning Point

• Andreas Kroitzsch
• An Introduction to the New Medicine

It was a November evening in 1989. The telephone rang; my sister who lived in Berlin called. "The border is open," she exclaimed with excitement. "The whole city has turned out. People are dancing on the wall! You have to turn on your TV immediately!"

I should mention that up until a few months before I had lived in West Berlin myself. I had spent my childhood and youth there and I had followed the news announcing the turning point. Did anybody really considered this revolution – and a soft one, too – possible?

And yet, despite the dramatic events happening in my hometown, the TV remained silent that evening. Because the book that I had started to read that afternoon had already caved in several walls inside myself. One of the very big mysteries of mankind was obviously on the brink of being resolved: the question of what actually makes us sick. And this turning point, as well, had been unimaginable for me until then. Did anybody really consider that possible?

I had already read some books, visited seminars and lectures, where people claimed that the causes for all diseases were found. They talked about disposition, heredity, and genetic code as well as unhealthy diets and all kinds of environmental influences, but also about weakened vitality, earth rays, and hidden allergies. Even more manifold were the therapies I encountered while I was studying to become an alternative practitioner. But the element that ultimately triggers a disease always remained in the dark.

The small book didn't just reveal the key to this secret to me. Also, my amazement about the one person who had been successful in putting together the many details and fragments was never-ending. And although Dr. Hamer still considered "disease" as something harmful or flawed at that time according to tradition – he would discover the biological "sense" only later on – the connections appeared so extraordinary, logical, and evident that from that November 9 on there was only one thing I wanted to do: to study the basics as soon as possible.

Some time later, I had gained modest first experiences in my work, and my family (the cat included) and I had also had some "ailments" which had been analyzed successfully.

So I set out to meet the discoverer of these connections in person. I met a man who possessed rich knowledge and who was a doctor with all his heart, concerned about the wellbeing of every single patient. Thus, I brought home from my visits not only new knowledge but also some unforgettable memories.

Dr. Hamer wrote several books and miscellanies that are indispensable for a comprehensive understanding of his findings. The following comments can and shall only offer an overview. Also, the limited space these pages offer doesn't allow dealing with all the different dimensions of the New Medicine; some of them have to remain unmentioned altogether.

15

Needless to say, I watched the pictures of the turning point in Berlin later on. At the same time, though, testimonials of a different turning point began to influence my day-to-day life. A new medical understanding arose that was growing every day and with every new personal experience. The perspective had changed and the parts of my former somewhat coherent medical worldview started to rearrange.

What Is a Disease?
- Cause
- Characteristics
- Meaningfulness

The core of the New Medicine (today: Germanic New Medicine®) consists of five laws, enabling us to define the development, the course, and the end of a disease. These laws include the cause, the characteristics, and the meaningfulness of what we call a "disease."

An increasing comprehension of these laws makes it more and more questionable, indeed, to stick to this traditional term. Nevertheless, we will stick to it for the time being to witness later on how its evaluation is changing due to a growing understanding.

In the light of Dr. Hamer's findings, the so-called diseases present themselves as processes that are initiated as soon as the creature – human or animal – is suddenly confronted with an obstacle.

First, Dr. Hamer observed that the beginning of a disease is always preceded by a dramatic experience of conflict. Second, he was able to prove that similar "diseases" always have the same conflict topic. Furthermore, he was able to find out where in the brain the control of the physical and psychological changes, which develop as a result of the conflict, is localized. Last, he proved that the processes in the brain, in the psyche, and in the organ take place simultaneously. The organic alteration, for example the growth of a tumor, comes to a halt after the conflict has been resolved.

Finally, he found out that all the organic alterations are not dysfunctions but regulation processes. What we call "diseases" are in fact *Meaningful Special Biological Programs*. From the first second on, such a program aims to overcome the exceptional conflict situation *psychologically*, by means of stress and increased and focused attention as well as *organically* via a meaningful alteration of a certain organ function.

On the basis of embryology, that is, the science of biological evolution, Dr. Hamer was able to show in detail how the organic regulation processes occur.

This last-mentioned discovery alone is so very ingenious and logical, that the heart of every physician and biologist who seriously considers it will jump for joy. This systematics also explains why the connections weren't discovered until now, because you can only understand them if you use the right key. If you have done that, however, a scientific field unfolds, the fascination of which is hardly to be surpassed.

Against this background, it seems no longer appropriate to try and plainly prevent or even eradicate diseases. The common understanding of "disease" as something bad, hostile, a threat from the outside (environment) or the inside (genetic make-up), as punishment, atonement, or the work of the devil has lost its foundation through these findings.

You could even go a step further. The world includes many different interests and life forms that cooperate and coexist; you have the wind, the weather, loss, and separation. As long as we cope with all these difficulties we are *healthy* in the true, superior sense.

The regulated course of the different special programs presents the normal status, which is ultimately designed to make the cooperation possible and to survive amidst all outside influences. Hence, it is normal and inevitable that we get "sick"; it means adapting to life, it is of service to us.

Psychosomatic Medicine and the New Medicine

• Disease Special Programs
• Terms of the New Medicine
• Analysis and Therapy

Consistent with the medical worldview, the medical psychosomatic medicine (psyche: soul, soma: body) considers diseases as defects. However, psychological conflicts and problems are regarded as their triggers. The "onset" of a disease occurs when the weakening of the organism exceeds a certain limit; in this case, the psychological strain is considered the last push, the straw that breaks the camel's back, the drop that spills the bucket.

Besides that, psychosomatic medicine also deals on different levels with the "meaning" of an illness, with the signals people send through their disease, how they communicate with their environment, what kind of personal developments and maturing processes they want to support unconsciously by being sick. But "disease" still is and remains an error in the system; it may be a welcome error, but it is always something harmful and, at times, "malignant."

So, how are we supposed to deal with "disease"? What can or should we do? Do the findings of the New Medicine make our entire understanding of "therapy" useless? After we found out which special program is taking place with a patient, should we leave it at that? Is it best to do nothing and patiently wait until things are "healed up"? Will future therapies mostly consist of finding resolutions for conflicts?

Before we turn to these questions, we want to look a little closer at the laws found by Dr. Hamer.

The Dirk Hamer Syndrome (DHS)

Every single special program, that is, what we have called "disease" so far, is triggered the same way. Dr. Hamer calls this law the "iron rule", which is to express that its course is valid in every single case without exception. The center of events is always a biological conflict. It initiates a program in the organism, which serves to overcome and resolve the very conflict.

The conflict always starts with a traumatic experience, the so-called "Dirk-Hamer-Syndrome" or DHS. Not every fright or every shock has the ability to trigger a biological conflict. Only if such an experience occurs unexpected and the person affected feels isolated because of it are the conditions met for a DHS, which marks the start of a special program; it is only then that a biological conflict exists.

The reader may find it hard to understand at this point that every cold or every diarrhea is supposed to be the result of a highly dramatic experience. But keep in mind that in a thunderstorm there is severe and less severe lightning in the sky, yet every single lightning fulfills the criteria necessary for its occurrence. Even the smallest, barely noticeable, electrical discharge has to be considered fully-fledged lightning, because it fulfills all the necessary conditions. There are severe and less severe Dirk Hamer Syndromes and even the mildest among them constitutes one if it fulfills all the criteria.

Biological

Dr. Hamer chose the term "biological conflict" wisely. It characterizes the common nominator of human and animal experience.

To give you an example, an animal can experience a "fear-of-death conflict" just like you and me. An animal feels fear of death if threatened, attacked, or driven into a corner. With us humans, a word, some news, or a deadly prognosis or diagnoses can also trigger this fear. The fear-of-death conflict is only one of about 150 biological conflicts listed in the "diagnosis table"; the number increases if we consider all the sub-forms.

A biological conflict has nothing to do with the widespread disease interpretations and –analogies. It is not to be understood in either a figurative or a spiritual sense; moreover, it can always be remembered by those affected as a concrete experience. The phrasing of the biological conflicts is very precisely chosen, so that it either matches individual cases – or it doesn't. If the affected person shakes his or her head and says, "That's not how it was", or "That's not how it felt", you have to continue with your search.

What kind of biological conflict an individual experiences in a particular situation is subjective – it depends on his or her social-, family-, and professional situation and also on conditioning and previous experiences. The biological conflict is not foreseeable, but it can always be retraced when the affected person tells his or her story.

"What Happened?"

In the beginning, there are usually certain symptoms – the so-called "ailments" –, or clinical findings, which are the result of an examination conducted because of the symptoms. It also happens that doctors find something, for instance, a changed blood level, by accident during a "routine checkup".

The first step is to estimate whether the underlying biological conflict is still active, or whether it has already been resolved. When did the symptoms start? Is the patient still experiencing them, or are they returning intermittently?

Oftentimes, the symptoms together with the narrowing down of the point of time lead directly to finding the conflict. If the experience is dating back a longer period of time, the search can prove to be a little more difficult.

The search for the conflict experience (DHS) is something the people involved do together. Only the affected person knows what happened and what he or she felt. The therapist or expert companion focuses on the correlation and the criteria in order to judge the experience in question regarding content, point of time, and intensity.

It is particularly advantageous to know the laws of the New Medicine even before you get "sick". In these cases, it doesn't take long to find the right, the associated conflict; from the first minute on, the affected person is "part of the process". But in all other cases you are by no means left in the dark either. The organic symptoms lead the way. The time of their occurrence, the diagnostic findings, and comparisons with earlier findings help to narrow down the point of time of the DHS. If you ask the affected person what happened after you finished this preparatory work, you have already narrowed down in your head the topic and the time of the event you are looking for.

This process requires heart, compassion, and cautiousness, not a schematic approach. Here are people who tell their stories, which are unique and filled with life. By communicating their stories, other people come close to us. In their stories you can feel evolvement, development, disappointment, and hurt feelings. Who would want to inquire about these things schematically?

The New Medicine is indeed so much more logical and systematic than the traditional medicine – there is hardly any computer freak around who, in view of the "diagnosis table", doesn't dream of a corresponding computer program. In its core, however, which consists of the affected people's stories, it requires applied intuition, openness, and human contact.

Oftentimes, a DHS initiates not just one but several special programs at the same time. An example: The statement of a spouse, "I am not sure if I really love you" can lead to a separation anxiety conflict (if the other one associates with that statement that he or she could be left right away), but also to a "nasty genital conflict" (if the statement is taken as a "blow below the belt"), or to a conflict of territory marking (if the affected person interprets the statement in the way that the other one is or could be attracted to a third person), to mention just a few possibilities. Every single one of these variations (and more) is possible alternatively but also at the same time.

Thus, the untrained observer can be presented with a conglomeration of symptoms, which makes it seem almost impossible to keep track. One symptom appears, another one disappears; then they both occur at the same time; a third one is added, and are we dealing with a new conflict?

However, the order in which the symptoms can occur as well as the possible combinations are by no means arbitrary. They happen according to certain biological rules.

What kind of conflicts we can actually suffer depends, among other things, on whether we are male or female, left- or right-handed, and also on the hormonal situation and on the active conflicts that already exist.

Furthermore, there are conflict constellations, the organic effects of which cancel each other out, so that there are no noticeable symptoms; and then there are circumstances under which such a deadlock can be cancelled again. And all of this can be put in order and be explained if you know the brain system and the Hamer Foci.

The Hamer Foci

At the same time a person experiences a conflict (DHS) and the organs start to be affected, a lesion appears in the brain, which is called a "Hamer Focus (HH).

In the cranial computed tomogram (CCT), these lesions are visible as concentric rings at the very location that is responsible for the relevant organ or function.

The "map" of the brain informs about the "Where is what". Every single switch point correlates on the one hand with a certain organ (a part or function of the organ respectively) and on the other hand with the appropriate biological conflict, so that you can conclude from the findings based on the CCT to the organic alteration as well as the conflict. In addition, every aspect of a conflict – provided that there are several – is individually existent in the brain. Thus, the CCT enables us to draw conclusions about the components of a conflict and the appropriate organic processes as well as to estimate the activity of the respective conflicts.

The CCT is part of the diagnostics and can't replace the anamnesis and the personal contact with the affected person in particular. It offers valuable clues in specific cases that turn out to be not clear enough. Dr. Hamer's literature provides a multitude of examples with the appropriate figures of the CT sections.

An Example

Let's assume a woman suffers a conflict when her doctor out of the blue after a routine checkup "breaks" to her the diagnosis of a severe, incurable disease. For our example we will disregard the question whether this diagnosis is right, and which criteria it is based upon. The patient, at least, accepts it as a reality and develops fear of death. From the moment this DHS occurred, cells of her lung tissue proliferate, leading to the development of nodules, a certain kind of lung tumors. These nodules grow as long as the conflict lasts. Once it is resolved, they stop growing.

This correlation is so clear that the reverse is permissible: If a patient has growing lung nodules, an active fear-of-death conflict exists at that point.

At the same time, a Hamer Focus (HH) appears in a specific location in the brain – in this case the brain stem -, which indicates through its characteristic occurrence that the conflict is active. If it were already resolved, the HH would present itself in a different way.

Synchrony

This leads us to another criterion. The progression of the conflict is synchronous to the progression of the alteration in the organ, and both, in turn, progress synchronously to the change of the Hamer Focus in the brain.

Thus, a severe conflict leads to a fast or severe alteration in the organ or the organ's function. A weaker active conflict has these alterations progress slowly.

However, in order to completely understand the principle of the three level's synchrony, we have to consider the fact that, principally, every special program has two phases, which differ from each other fundamentally. For, it is these two phases in particular that progress on all three levels – psyche, brain, and organ – synchronously.

To come to the point, we practically never noticed these two phases until now. If you have understood the New Medicine, however, you can't overlook them any more!

The first phase begins as soon as the conflict arises and is thus called the "conflict active phase". It is characterized by a specific reaction to an unexpected conflict situation in two respects. First, the creature suffering a conflict reacts with its entire vegetative nervous system in a typical way. And second, specific organic or functional alterations appear, which are directly connected to the content of the conflict and, therefore, vary for case to case.

The Vegetative Course

Let us first consider the general vegetative reaction. Everybody knows how it feels to experience an unexpected, dramatic situation that is threatening.

The intellect revolves around the experience – in our case the shock of the diagnosis – and tries out resolutions by way of thinking; however, it oftentimes goes in circles.

The people relive the situation again and again, but that doesn't help. They are caught inside themselves; they can't communicate their feelings. They don't have an appetite and their sleep is interrupted; they fall asleep thinking of the conflict and they wake up in the morning thinking of it.

If a conflict remains unresolved for a longer period of time, the weight loss shows and the lack of sleep is increasingly obvious. The body seems emaciated, the complexion is pale, and the hands are cold. Other people say, "You don't look well".

However, there is usually no genuine feeling of being sick. People do feel stressed or overstrung but not really sick. This is the first phase of a special program also called the "conflict active phase".

The second phase is the resolution- or healing phase. It begins with the resolution of the conflict – provided that it will be resolved. As soon as the object of the conflict becomes superfluous, the vegetative nervous system switches over into vagotony (relaxation). The "resolved conflict phase" begins and it can be considered the compensation for the previous stress phase.

The obsessive dealing with the conflict stops completely. People develop an appetite again and gain weight quickly. Former sleeping problems are now replaced by a deep and relaxing sleep. The complexion isn't pale any more and the hands are warm. Fatigue and lack of energy are predominant, which can reach a state of exhaustion. Now, the patients say," I feel sick"; they are worried because climbing the stairs tires them out, or because they are physically not strong enough to do the gardening.

But how different is the experience for people who know the New Medicine! They know that their conflict is resolved. They even know exactly what kind of conflict it was and they understand their physical condition as the necessary phase of recovery after exhausting work. In addition, they can estimate the anticipated duration of this phase of exhaustion and respond accordingly. The people around them who also understand can support them during that process instead of reacting with fear, pity, or even feelings of guilt.

The Organic Course

Besides this general vegetative level, the two phases of a special program – a "disease" – always have another specific level, which is determined by the kind of the respective special program, that is, by the conflict content. A specific organic or functional alteration occurs. In the case of the fear-of-death conflict described above it is the growing of lung nodules during the conflict active phase.

In order to understand the "correlation" of the organic symptoms and the individual conflicts, we remember that our special programs also occur in animals and that these are archaic functions that have been in existence for eons.

The original archaic fear of death in humans is connected with the idea of suffocating. Whenever we feel fear of death, our body still reacts as if we would suffocate – no matter what the concrete incidence that led to the fear of death.

The special program triggered by fear of death consists of extending the inner surface of the lung to be able to use more breathing air. This is accomplished by increasing the lung tissue. In doing so, the (alleged) lack of breathing air is to be compensated.

Like the absorption of breathing air that is to be increased in the case of fear of death, the same applies, for example, for the absorption of food in the adenous parts of the digestive system. Today, some of the special programs are not directly comprehensible for us any longer, because, in the meantime, humans have developed other forms of essential "food lumps" like money, stocks, or property shares. Nevertheless, we can grasp the original sense of all these programs through our comprehension even today.

Very often, the organic alterations that take place during the conflict active phase aren't noticed. Only when the second phase sets in with fatigue and the feeling of being sick after solving the conflict do organic symptoms often appear as well. For, from the moment of the conflict resolution the organic or functional alteration isn't necessary any longer; it has become superfluous. Now, the organism begins the repairing, which is associated with edema (buildup of fluids), swelling, inflammation, and often also with pain. In the healing phase, the brain, as well, develops an edema in the location of the Hamer Focus, which has more or less severe effects depending on its position and intensity.

In our example, the excess cells in the lung tissue, which were useful until then, are catabolized again in the healing phase. If that is not possible, the nodules are at least encapsulated. If patients know about the connections, they can prepare themselves for the specific physical effects they have to expect and to deal with based on the previous conflict.

The First Symptoms

The *conflict active* phase leads only in few cases to the affected person seeking help from a therapist; the isolating component prevails and the person feels more efficient and able to work under pressure than usual because of the overall sympathicotonic state. In addition, there are often no or only few physical symptoms. As mentioned above, the symptoms don't start until the conflict is resolved, which is then also the time the person seeks medical help.

The ability to understand the symptoms of the healing phase by means of the New Medicine doesn't change the fact that the person feels sick during that phase.

Depending on the case, a fever, pain, prolonged weakness, and organic symptoms of all kinds can appear more or less severely and persistently.

Being aware that it is "only" the healing phase doesn't change the fact that those affected have to go through this phase of the disease, and that it can push them in some cases, depending on the case history, to their physical and psychological limits. It goes without saying that, besides compassion and compassion, the patients should receive the best possible medical care in order to ease their discomfort.

Often, the treatment of a "disease" begins at a time when the healing has already started, and the most severe diagnoses are also made at that time.

The example of the patient who developed fear of death because of a threatening diagnosis wasn't chosen accidentally. In the traditional medicine, such a diagnosis (possibly with an included prognosis) is in most cases considered the "truth" and the patient experiences it as such. And with many people who start searching for their conflicts by means of the New Medicine, the shock of the diagnosis is very often predominant and is accompanied by even more dramatic effects than the original conflict, the effects of which had led the patient to see a doctor.

The Ontogenetic System

People who take their first steps to get into the matter are confronted with the same problems Dr. Hamer encountered at the time he began to match the physical symptoms with the biological conflicts. The big difference is, of course, that Dr. Hamer entered new scientific territory, while today we "just" have to find our way in the system he discovered.

The initial confusion is the following: In one case (like in our example) a tumor grows in the *conflict active phase*. In other cases (a kidney cyst, for instance), however, this growth doesn't occur until the healing phase.

A biliary colic always occurs after the *resolution* of a conflict whereas a speech impediment or palsy develops shortly after the *DHS*. Or, in other words: In many clinical pictures the symptoms do not occur until the conflict has been resolved. The secret why the different kinds of tissue behave so fundamentally contrary to each other lies in their embryologic origin.

All cells and tissue structures in our organisms (as well as in animal organisms) stem from one of three so-called germ layers. In the first days of the embryonic stage, these layers are still clearly organized, but during the further progression and growth they develop into the complex organism that humans are through manifold and highly complicated foldings. Embryology provides information about which cell structure or which organ originated from which germ layer.

Each of the three germ layers is associated with a group of conflicts and these conflicts differ fundamentally from each other.

First, there are conflicts that concern the direct survival, that is, purely existential conflicts. The fear-of-death conflict mentioned above belongs to this group. Second, there are conflicts connected with the intactness of the organism, with inner and outer stability and the performance. The "collapse of self-esteem" is among the conflicts of this category. And the third, large, group consists of all those conflicts, which develop in encounters with other individuals. They deal with areas like setting boundaries, separation, safety, hierarchy, and rivalry.

These three groups are, in turn, associated each with one part of our brain where the respective Hamer Foci appear as well. The brain stem controls the organs of the inner germ layer (endoderm), the cerebral cortex those of the outer germ layer (ectoderm), and the white matter and the cerebellum are responsible for the groups of the middle germ layer.

And while tissue cells of the ectoderm *die* during the conflict phase, the tissue of the endoderm *develops* additional cells during that same phase. The latter are catabolized again in the healing phase – mostly by means of swelling and inflammation – while the ectodermal tissue develops new cells during that same phase.

The classification of the so-called diseases according to germ layers is the key to a consistent and self-contained system. And together with the psyche level and the brain level, a fascinating picture arises that includes the entire medical science.

The knowledge of the ontogenetic system makes it possible to estimate the course of a special program in each individual case. If the conflict is known, the symptoms that will develop after its resolution in the second phase are basically predictable. As mentioned above, many symptoms don't occur until this phase, which means that the risk of complications is here the highest.

The patients can be prepared for what they have to expect, and necessary preparations can be made for possible complications.

Conflict Active- or Healing Phase?

It is of utmost importance to differentiate whether a symptom belongs to the conflict- or to the healing phase. One would think that this would already result from the vegetative overall situation: if the human being is in the state of relaxation (vagotony) the appropriate symptoms can be attributed to the healing phase.

In principle, that is right, but it doesn't turn out to be that clear all the time. Even during a resolution, another conflict can be active, so that the outcome is a "mixed form." It is essential to exactly differentiate in every case, and the ontogenetic system is the basis to do that.

Not only the kind of symptoms but also their anticipated *intensity* as well as the approximate *duration* of the healing phase can be estimated. In this context, it is useful to have a look at the "conflict mass", which, in turn, can be estimated from the duration and the intensity of the previous conflict.

These values are, of course, only rough estimates and are subject to fluctuations resulting from the everyday life and the overall situation of those affected and, thus, an estimate is always a snapshot, which is geared to the past.

This estimate also concerns the "epileptoid crisis", which, in simple terms, marks the switchover point in the brain from the buildup of the edema to its expulsion. At least with the conflicts controlled by the cerebrum, it presents the most critical moment in the course of the healing phase.

Every special program has its characteristic crisis. The anticipated intensity depends on what was stated above concerning the conflict mass. The time of its occurrence, however, can be predicted quite accurately if the time of the conflict resolution is known. And regarding the question whether a conflict should be resolved, it is important to always keep in mind the anticipated intensity of the epileptoid crisis.

Knowing Instead of Believing

Nobody has to believe in the New Medicine, because it takes place inside every one of us and with the necessary basic knowledge you can experience it with your own body and in your own soul. Besides the necessary clarity, it also increases trust if the affected people are successful in finding the conflicts that caused their diagnosis and symptoms. In the run-up, they read something, comprehended it, and now they are experiencing that what they read is true – with their own body and with all characteristics; they have become one of the people who know. That can leave them beyond many a doubt, much more than well-meaning words could have done.

At this point at the latest it becomes clear that the New Medicine isn't a "method" patients can choose to be treated with like with other so-called "procedures" we have been used to up until now.

The active participation of the patient is necessary from the first minute on. Even more: patients and expert companions are a team, only able to work if both have understood what all of this is about. If the patients haven't internalized at least the basics of the New Medicine, they won't be able to grasp its importance, let alone to apply it to their particular situation. In other words: If people seek help in the New Medicine without knowing about the basic connections just hoping for an effective therapy, they will walk this path in vain.

Dr. Hamer always emphasizes that "the patient is the boss of the process", and that can be taken literally, because, in the end, the patients have to take the sole responsibility for their decisions and will have to deal with the resulting consequences. Thus, it is their right to get as much information as possible and to thoroughly evaluate the respective situation. Not persuasion, but help and support are appropriate here.

We are now experiencing something in the medical field that has been a matter of course in psychology and psychotherapy for a long time: Responsibility is returned to the patient who is considered an independently thinking and acting individual. Sure, it isn't always easy to carry this responsibility yourself. It is a continuous exercise for both sides – and at the same time a great chance. Many of our relationships suffer from just that, one person feeling responsible for the other, or being pushed into feeling that way.

Theme With Variations

With the presentation of the two phases and their chronology, we have been introduced to the basic model. Nature acts out this model in many different ways, so that in practice, that is, in everyday life, we are confronted with new variations of this basic pattern all the time.

First, it has to be mentioned that many – although not all – people remember the moment they resolved a conflict as precise as the moment of shock when it emerged. There are conflicts that resolve little by little over a longer time period, but often the conflict resolution (conflictolysis, CL) is a defined moment. It is the switchover point from the stress phase (sympathicotonia) to the relaxation phase (vagotony).

Now, what are the possible variations regarding the basic two-phase model? We get an idea if we look at the abundance of clinical pictures listed in our medical textbooks and reference books.

There are diseases that appear suddenly and disappear again in the foreseeable future. Others turn into chronic diseases that can last for years, or even for a whole lifetime. Others, again, start slowly and develop sometimes severe and then again less severe symptoms. Certain groups of diseases are characterized by continuous organic matter degradation, others by inflammation and pain. Diseases that appear and disappear again and again are classified as "relapsing", the symptom-free intervals lasting for days or even years. Some of them always occur in certain situations, for instance while being in contact with animals, or on vacation.

The general rule is: The course of the symptoms has to match the course of the conflict. If a symptom recurs intermittently, there must be situations in which the relevant conflict is *activated* again and again. This, in turn, applies only if the relevant symptom belongs to the conflict active phase (for example, angina pectoris). However, should the recurring symptom be part of the healing phase (e.g., neurodermatitis), it will always appear after the *resolution* of a conflict relapse, or in situations that provide a temporary short-term resolution for an existing conflict.

The Resolution

What has to happen before a resolution actually sets in? Considering all the differences of the possible conflicts, there are three basic aspects of a resolution: outer event, inner awareness, and individual acting.

Apparently, some conflicts resolve through an outer event alone: The cat that was missing walks into the door, or the opponent offers his hand in reconciliation. Other situations are resolved as people realize something that helps them to reevaluate, for instance, by becoming aware of their own feelings and motivations that led to the conflict. The "reevaluation" of a diagnosis in the light of the New Medicine can belong here as well. Other conflicts can be resolved as people make a decision and act accordingly.

There are always all three components existent, but the emphases and, thus, the possibilities are different in each case. An act – for example as a result of the active inner dealing with the topic – can help us realize things. And the outer event becomes effective only if we realize its meaning.

It is least reliable to wait for an external change or an internal realization. The best and most effective things for the affected people are those they themselves can do and attempt in order to directly – by acting – or at least indirectly – by dealing with it inwardly - resolve their conflict.

Conflict Resolution – Not Always

It may appear from the previous statements that the *resolution* is the only way, or just the best way for nature to deal with a biological conflict.

The New Medicine enables us to gain deep insight into the way life has provided for its own continuity for millions of years. And not only that: We discover ourselves as parts of a system that optimizes itself continuously. Thanks to the code within us that controls our special programs, we actually exist *during every moment in the greatest possible stability* in relation to the things that befall us from the outside.

As soon as it is no longer possible or even meaningful that a conflict is resolved - for example, if the accumulated conflict mass has become too extensive - the organism immediately uses a second- or third-best version. And, thus, you can find every imaginable variety and version and every possible combination between the "active" and the "resolved" conflict.

The first, basic, version is that of the conflict not being resolved but alleviated in one way or the other and continuing to exist. In the second version, the effects of one conflict are reduced by adding another one. We will return to that version later.

The Hanging Conflict

Some conflicts in everyday life can't be resolved even if there is reasonable time. Many an insult goes so deep, many a relationship is that hopeless that there is no direct resolution in sight. Many people suffer quietly and can't find a way out. Others don't have the means to free themselves from an emergency.

The path nature chooses in these cases to secure the survival is the "hanging conflict". Such a conflict isn't resolved, but it has lost its immediate drama. People come to terms with the status quo. These hanging conflicts with all their different versions constitute most of the cases.

A hanging conflict is "hanging" because it is being activated again and again. Strictly speaking, conflict active- and healing phases alternate at frequent intervals. The physical symptoms occur according to the sequence of the phases. If the stress phases outbalance, we talk about "hanging activity". If the healing phases are in the foreground, the term "hanging resolution" is more appropriate. In addition, there are conflicts that occur intermittently, are resolved, and recur. They are called relapsing conflicts, and on the organic level we are dealing with the relapsing diseases or disorders.

If a symptom occurs, which, according to the ontogenetic system, belongs to the healing phase - for example pain in the shoulder joint – it doesn't necessarily mean that the conflict is resolved. It can also be part of a hanging resolution, which means, strictly speaking, that the conflict is not resolved. Hence, it is always important to find out whether the definite resolution has actually taken place. Has the inner view regarding the conflict content changed fundamentally? What happened? Has the experience been positive and relieving? How does the overall vegetative situation present itself in the before/after comparison? How is the person's appetite, need for sleep, and inner calmness?

As long as a hanging conflict isn't resolved, there is no foreseeable end to the activity – and also no end to the symptoms. Nevertheless, the fact mentioned above saying that not every conflict can be resolved creates a dilemma at times. In those cases, the creativity of everybody involved is needed. However, people also realize the limits with regard to the things that can be done depending on the possibilities of the affected people within their familial and social system.

The Tracks

The question comes to mind, what is it that activates hanging or relapsing conflicts again and again, what keeps them "alive". Sometimes the answer is obvious. It is easy to imagine that someone whose bank has axed his or her funds is reminded of the conflict every time he or she pulls out the wallet. And an employee who feels bullied in the office more than likely suffers a conflict relapse every time she runs into the respective co-worker; maybe it already happens as soon as she enters the building. It wouldn't be surprising either if she didn't experience any conflicts and, thus, any symptoms after work, on the weekends, or during her vacation.

Such a dimension of the conflict, which puts the patient internally "on the train" to the overall conflict, is called a "track". These tracks can be as manifold as life itself and they are always immediately connected with the DHS. After identifying the DHS, the next piece of the puzzle that has to be traced is finding the tracks. But, after all, the "hot trail" has already been found. Every track patients can identify for themselves brings them closer to adequately handle their conflict.

For they know now what they are suffering from, they localized the conflict, and if they also know the associated tracks applying for them, they can start watching themselves.

An affected person will realize that his ringing in the ears increases whenever he is in the same room with the person who is part of his *"hearing conflict"*. A patient will find that the diarrhea actually occurs after his partner has returned safely from a meeting with her ex-husband, that is, after the resolution of the recurring *"undigested anger"* (even if it originally concerned a completely different partner).

Or another patient will observe, how the lump at her neck is swelling temporarily every time the *"frontal fear"* triggered by the medical diagnosis that she "has only three more months to live" flares up and disappears again.

Fragments of Memory

What is the nature of the tracks? We all know the phenomenon that we can exactly remember the details of the situation even years and decades after the dramatic conflict experience. Not only can we exactly reproduce the spoken words, we also inwardly hear the sound and the tone of the voice; we know where we were sitting or standing, or the ring tone of the telephone.

A smell that was in the air at that time – maybe a certain meal was prepared or a cake was made – can suddenly take us back to the emotions of that situation.

A certain particular characteristic of our partner might trigger an "allergic reaction", because we experienced this posture, this movement, or this noise in a dramatic context with another person.

The largest part of this sensory imprint our brain produces of the situation at the time of the DHS remains unaware to us. We actually store with all our available senses – the sense of sight, hearing, smell, taste, touch, and balance and temperature – a complete hologram of our internal and external perception and keep this image in the depths of our brain. This can go to such length that people suddenly remember details of a difficult conflict situation although they hadn't even learned to walk at that time.

In this context, psychologists talk about "traumatic memory" when it comes to traumatic experiences, and they found that the individual memory aspects are filed separately in the brain. Therefore - contrary to the "normal" memory - if an individual aspect appears, we don't remember automatically the entire sequence of the experience, but the aspect and the associated emotions remain isolated. This way, we don't have to relive the traumatic, overwhelming situation internally over and over again.

However, it looks very much as if this was also a part of our brain's learning strategy. We learn to perceive the very first signs of a possibly dangerous situation and to act accordingly, so that we don't have to relive a situation internally – by remembering – or externally – by experiencing it again. Our brain virtually warns us with every single "symptom" against falling into the trap again and most of the time we are not even aware of it.

That way, even those conflicts that are basically dealt with can continue to "cook on a low heat" or flare up again and again if just one single track remains; for example, if you drive only sporadically by the company building you worked in until the sudden layoff, or if you hear only once in a while the noise of an airplane flying over the house, which, unconsciously, activates the panic you lived through as a child during an air strike.

You don't even have to consciously hear the plane; the Hamer Focus is nonetheless activated and the organic alteration takes place, which, then, presents itself through recurring ailments. Practically every experience and every sensation can turn into a track: a separation, a spoken word, a dripping faucet, a certain kind of food or a smell, but also pollen, cat hair particles, or a certain noise frequency.

Thus, an "allergic reaction" is not a sensitivity of the body regarding a certain substance, but a short conflict relapse with subsequent resolution. It is triggered by a perception that reminds us of the original DHS. And this perception usually happens unconsciously.

The Alleviated Conflict

But what a chance presents itself if we can become aware of these tracks! On the one hand, it will be possible to deal with the conflict mentally and to put it into perspective. On the other hand, it enables patients to do something – which, in turn, encourages them to take action where, before, they felt like victims. This is an enormous asset when it comes to self-healing. She can choose a different route in the city and he can consciously take the plane to go on vacation in order for all his senses to experience the differences between the current planes and those from 1944. In other words: Patients can begin to alleviate or "downtransform" their conflict.

Each situation is different and overall resolution suggestions don't lead anywhere. The best suggestions and ideas are those developed by the affected people. And in the very best case they themselves can start taking action and do something to heal.

The Sublimated Conflict

As indicated before, in addition to the model of the "hanging" conflict there is a second version our organism uses in order to exist with an unresolved – or unsolvable – conflict. It is based on the fact that the brain can create "constellations" of several conflicts, with which their characteristics and effects can be seriously changed.

This second version can't be explained here in detail, because it would go beyond the scope of this introduction. However, it is an extremely important factor without which a comprehension of the New Medicine, particularly for the individual case, is not possible. And here, at the latest, a place at the "round table" of the New Medicine becomes available for those who professionally deal with the human psyche – and who might have two objections. First, not every psychologically burdened patient is physically sick. And, second, the categorization into biological conflicts isn't enough to appropriately describe the map of the psyche.

To say just this: Two or more Hamer Foci, respectively, can be in constellation with each other. At the same time, though, not every possible combination is a constellation. The latter have fundamentally different effects depending on the category.

Some constellations lead to the largely or complete neutralizing of the organic alterations of both conflicts involved. The conflict mass accumulated up to that point is virtually frozen. Thus, a conflict, although it persists, can be clinically "mute" for years and decades if it exists in one of the mentioned constellations.

On the psychological level, the conflicts involved are *sublimated*. The concrete conflict content takes a back seat and the experience now forms our behaviour, our thinking and our imagination on a new level.

This presents an insight into the broad field of psychological problems to the point of the so-called mental and emotional disorders. The constellations, particularly those of the cerebrum, are to be considered "super-special programs": The sum of the individual parts results in something new. And in each of these superior programs you can recognize a similar "super-meaning". But that is only the beginning of this exciting chapter. A large part of what constitutes our character to the point of preferences and abilities, creativity, intuition, or the "seventh sense" can be attributed to early conflict experiences that were sublimated in constellations.

Conflicts—Parts of Life

Here, at the latest, it becomes clear that the negative overtone of the word "conflict" basically doesn't do it justice. It should be sensed value-free and its resolution is only one among several equal alternatives.

If you read about Dr. Hamer's discovery in the media, you usually come across a passage that reads for instance like this: "Hamer claims you just have to resolve the conflict and the cancer is cured."

After what has been said so far, there is no need to further comment on the simplification and distortion inherent in this statement. For, the primary purpose is not to heal cancer, but more so to recognize it for what it is, which automatically results in possible ways for a healing. But just as "cancer" isn't a disease per se, the patient can't be categorized as sick, because he or she has a conflict!

Conflicts are a part of the natural course of life. Each of us has to deal perpetually with small, bigger, hanging, or resolved conflicts. We even saw that conflicts can stabilize health in certain constellations! So, you should be careful when people tell you that health equals being free of conflicts, and with the help of the New Medicine you can and should finally realize such a state.

And if a person even claims to cure "cancer" or other diseases through "reprogramming", he or she hasn't understood a single thing. If we start meddling with conflicts instead of symptoms, as we have done up to now, nothing is gained.

It also isn't part of a "conflict anamnesis" according to the New Medicine to identify or even deal with every existing conflict, particularly those of infantile and early nature. Dr. Hamer's findings don't help us to become "doers".

If you work with them, however, you will be amazed over and over again by the wisdom, the variety, and the ingenuity inherent in our organism, which, in many cases, decides for itself whether a conflict will be resolved, persists, or will be alleviated. We are not able to influence that with our thinking. It is best for us to think things *through*, observe, and give our advice and support. What we can contribute besides knowledge and experience are, above all, our own enthusiasm and candidness. We shouldn't hesitate either to admit openly if there is something we don't know.

Life wouldn't be what it is if every situation was solvable, or if there was always a way out. The New Medicine isn't a universal remedy, a tool to gain control over life. It shines a light both on the possibilities and on the limits of life on earth. It doesn't just show how life works, but also how it can end. Thus, it calls on us to pay attention to that aspect as well, whether we are companions or patients. And who among us isn't at some point a "patient" in this regard?

The Responsible Patient

There is no specific method of therapy based on the New Medicine. The focus is always on the understanding the patients gain about their situation. This knowledge enables them to actively take action, which is the therapy in its true sense.

It then depends on the circumstance which "methods" should be chosen to support them medically. In one case surgery may be necessary, in another case it's a matter of symptomatic treatment, of strengthening certain organs, revulsion, or building up the muscles.

It can be discussed whether this is achieved by means of phytotherapy in one case, or with thorn therapy in another. Thus, many a naturopathic procedure is rather the "background music" for the real therapy, and the valid question arises, how much "procedure" is actually necessary considering that many of these procedures were originally developed against something that now turns out to be meaningful.

Therefore, at least a critical re-evaluation is necessary. A lot of patients don't want to take too many drugs, because they are of the opinion that their organism can help itself.

It's another thing, though, if we talk about methods that can be used to avoid complications, for example, to alleviate the symptoms of the healing phase or the epileptoid crisis.

The spouse or partner, the children, parents, and friends are as much part of the patients' system as the attending doctors and therapists. The patients' freedom of action is determined by the external circumstances, their social and financial situation, as much as by their self-confidence, inner stability, fears, courage, and their willingness to take risks.

The more support they get (or have got) from their families and their system, the earlier they will be able to make unconventional decisions.

Or, in other words: A decision becomes difficult or impossible if those affected are internally or externally out on a limb. Hence, the patients should include the people who support them as much as possible in their process. This also applies to the attending doctor or the family doctor. A skeptic or "enemy" can turn into an ally and supporter if he or she gets a real chance to become involved.

The real therapy is the one that patients themselves bring about based on their understanding and acting. The motivation grows with everything they do as a result of that understanding, even with every relapse they observe and understand.

As a matter of fact, nothing works *without* motivation. Thus, we see patients who come to their next visit with a number of new tracks they discovered in the meantime. And we see the glow in their eyes when they say," I remembered another thing."

We are dealing with people who, instead of filling files with their medical history, suddenly create diagrams showing their history "according to Hamer". And they point with their index finger to a gap in the list and say," This is something I have yet to figure out. Something is missing here." Those are the responsible patients. They can't be fooled any more.

The 5 Biological Laws of the New Medicine in Their Exact Wording

1. The "Iron Rule of Cancer" with three criteria:

    1.1. Every Meaningful Biological Special Program (SBS) originates from a DHS (Dirk-Hamer-Syndrome), i.e., from a very severe, highly acute, dramatic, and isolating conflict shock, which occurs on three levels simultaneously: in the psyche, the brain, and the organ.

    1.2. In the moment of the DHS, the biological conflict determines both the location of the SBS in the brain (the so-called Hamer Focus) and the location of the cancer or cancer-equivalent disease in the organ.

    1.3. The development of the SBS on all three levels (psyche, brain, organ) from the DHS to the conflict resolution (conflictolysis, CL) and the epileptic/epileptoid crisis at the peak of the PCL phase (healing phase) as well as the return to normal (normotony) runs synchronously.

2. The Law of the Two Phases of all Meaningful Biological Special Programs (SBS) provided that there is a conflict resolution (CL).

3. The Ontogenetic System of the Meaningful Biological Special Programs (SBS) of Cancer and Cancer-equivalent Diseases (cancer SBS and cancer-equivalent SBS)

4. The Ontogenetic System of the Microbes

5. Every so-called disease has to be comprehended as part of a Meaningful Biological Special Program of nature (which need to be understood in the context of evolution).

Andreas Kroitzsch, October 2005

Conflicts and Resolutions
• Examples from the practice

Like in the first volume of the factor-L series, we compiled again examples from the practice in order to make the introduction to Dr. Hamer's New Medicine and the understanding of the processes easier for you. This time, however, we edited the stories. Instead of the original interviews, you will find retold experiences on the following pages. The cases as such are authentic. They were, however, made into short stories and edited accordingly. The stories are told in such a way that the triggers (Dirk Hamer syndromes [DHS]) of the Meaningful Special Biological Programs (SBS), which are called diseases in the traditional medicine, are being emphasized, so that they are easily comprehensible.

In doing so, we want to clarify that conflicts are perceived in a very personal way. Consequently, there are no triggers that always and in every person lead to a DHS. Things that throw us off balance today may not even make us stagger tomorrow. In turn, the infamous drop that spills the bucket can well hit us with a DHS, or, according to the traditional medicine, make us sick.

If you have ever seen a boxing match with a lot of blows being exchanged, you can easily comprehend the process. The fighters can stomach a blow in the first round quite well, because they feel strong and are in good condition. But if they receive the same blow several rounds later after they were hit repeatedly, it can lead to a knockout even if it is carried out with only half the power.

The amount of hits can reduce our resisting power in all life situations enormously. A seemingly minor conflict that strikes us according to the known criteria (existential – unexpected – isolating) can trigger a DHS if it worsens our overall personal situation. Those are the all too well known situations that have us think, "That's all I need right now" or "That's the last thing I needed".

The following reports clearly show that every individual perceives a conflict as existential depending on the situation and on his or her very personal perception. These experiences are supposed to enable you to recognize your very own conflict triggers and (if possible/necessary) to resolve the conflicts.

A Friendly Turn

• Kathrin and the allergies

"I see," said Kathrin and had a skeptical look around. If she said that and said it the way she just did, Bert knew that it meant pure panic. However, he had to admit that he, too, was surprised. That was not how he had imagined Klaus and Marion's apartment. He scratched the back of his head in shock. "And what kind of a hole is this?" Tom asked. "If even Tom notices it, I obviously see right", thought Bert and scratched his head again.

Tom was twelve years old and a slob like no other. Tom decided to tidy up only after they had gone through the three-step program.

Step 1: Constant requests to finally tidy up with subsequent threats of punishment by Bert.
Step 2: Ignoring of the requests and threats by Tom.
Step 3: Punishment, angry yelling, and tidying up.

Previously, it had even been a five-step plan, but in the meantime, Bert had found the right punishment: Tom simply wasn't allowed to watch the game of his favourite team. He went through that only three times before he caved.

"Are you sure we shouldn't to go to a hotel after all?" asked Kathrin and was already turning to the door.

"Not really," Bert admitted. "But see how late it is. This hick town has just one small hotel. And I am sure that they already closed for the day." Kathrin looked at her watch. Then she sighed, turned again, sighed again, and had obviously made a decision. "Well, guys, then tidying up it is. If we all help, it can't be that bad." A look around in the kitchen made her sigh a third time. "Although...maybe it can."

During the following two hours the three of them scrubbed, wiped, and tidied up as best they could. They vacuum-cleaned and dusted. That worked out fine; the next house was ten meters away and the neighbours across the street didn't complain either. After all, 10:00 p.m. wasn't the most convenient time to do that kind of work.

Tom came across an abandoned-looking cat while he was cleaning, and later on he also found three young kittens. After the cleaning crew had already filled three bags of garbage, Kathrin found some cat food as well. Greedily, the living room tigers jumped at the food. "Since when do Klaus and Marion have cats anyway? Couldn't they have mentioned them at least?" Kathrin asked. Bert shrugged his shoulders. He fought with a very persistent dirt crust at the fridge. "And they are your friends?" complained Tom. "You better not gripe again when I invite Dirk. He isn't half the dirt bag."

Bert was worried when Kathrin didn't answer. It was proof that his wife had experienced a severe shock. He couldn't even understand it himself yet. He looked at her anxiously. Kathrin was wiping the hallway in disgust. And she was sniffing. Her eyes were swollen and she wheezed over and over again as if she couldn't breathe. Bert sighed and turned to the freezer again. If only he had known...

Actually, they just wanted to relax for a week. For, even if the hick town really was just a hick town, it was the ideal place to relax. It was a wonderful area and, in addition, it was remote. The few inhabitants here were friendly and Bert wanted to take his time and finally go on a real fishing trip again. Kathrin just needed a book, sun, and water. And Tom brought his surfboard. He appreciated the privacy the place offered, because he didn't have any experience with it yet. Klaus and Marion had offered them to spend the week in their small house while they were on an author tour.

"Maybe we should have had a look at the house beforehand," Bert thought angrily. It looked much bigger on the photo, but that wasn't the worst. "We should have asked for inside photos. Then we would have decided to stay at the hotel right away." Angrily, he took an empty glass out of the fridge – well, it was almost empty. Something hairy was growing in it. "I wouldn't be surprised if that hairy something jumped out and shouted Buh!," Bert thought in disgust and threw it in the garbage.

He couldn't stop thinking about Klaus and Marion. How could he and Kathrin be so wrong about them? They always appeared so attractive and well groomed and they had had very good conversations with them. They had been in Bert and Kathrin's city for two weeks. They had met them in a bar and had invited them to their place.

He had considered their offer generous. And although he didn't really want to live in someone else's house, he agreed this time without hesitating. "How stupid of you," he was swearing at himself inwardly. "Now you know why they have been so generous."

Meanwhile, Tom and Kathrin had given up swearing. Tom mumbled between his lips something like "stupid idea." But that was all they were able to say. They were sitting on the dingy couch, exhausted. The living room sparkled, and so did the hallway and the bedroom. And the kitchen was almost finished as well. They still had to do the bathroom, which would take them at least another half hour.

Half an hour after midnight, an exhausted Bert and Kathrin lay next to each other on the extendable couch. Kathrin was relieved that she had brought their sheets. She was particular about that. "And rightfully so," she thought, feeling confirmed. Her nose was running worse than in the afternoon, everything was blocked, the eyes were itchy and she was sneezing constantly. "As if this isn't enough, I got a head cold on top of everything," she grumbled and sniffed in her handkerchief. She looked at Bert with runny eyes. He ran his hand over her hair. "Honey, if I didn't know better, I would think that you have an allergic cold. " Then he looked around, saw the cats, and added, "Or that you are allergic to cats."

Tom had spread a blanket on the floor and had built himself something like a bed on it. He was already asleep. The cats scattered around the rooms, purring contentedly. "They don't have anything to eat, everything is spoilt," he growled before he fell asleep. "Tomorrow morning we'll leave as quickly as possible," Kathrin remarked. "And we might as well take a plane south. There is no way that I stay here."

The next morning they had a look at their work and were satisfied. It wasn't even 6:00 a.m. The house didn't seem any more comfortable – still everything looked a little shabby and tired - but at least it was clean now. Tom had disposed of the garbage and, astonishingly, didn't even complain. "More than likely he's too tired," thought Bert. All three of them looked at the cats thoughtfully. The big one had already filled her belly and the three little ones just had their second helping. They seemed starved.

"Do you think they asked someone to feed the cats? And to clean the litter box?" Tom muttered. On an empty stomach, that hadn't been the highlight of the morning for the boy. Anyhow, it wasn't as bad any more as it had been last night before they cleaned the bath when it had seemed as though nobody had taken care of the dirt for days. "The poor creatures," Bert thought, but he pulled back his hand when the mother cat pressed her head against it.

"Hey, they are really clean," said Kathrin. "Although that is the only thing that is clean in this house. That was clean!" she corrected herself in the next moment. Bert seemed undecided. "Shall we leave them here?" he asked his wife. "What if nobody is taking care of them?" She shrugged her shoulders. "What are we supposed to do with them? We can only leave them enough food and water."

"I would at least open the window a little bit, so that they can get out if they have to, mom. Really, you can't leave them locked up here like that. I don't think these dirt bags asked someone to check on the cats. I am sure they thought that we'd do it," Tom piped up. Bert tapped him on the shoulders in agreement. "I am thinking the same, son. Let's improvise something." With that, they walked over to the kitchen window.

Half an hour later, that was done as well. Using a sock (half-clean, as Bert had suspiciously noticed before), they had fixed the window in a way that it opened about ten centimeters. In between, they put a wooden block Tom had found outside. The cats were very quick to understand what that was about. Five minutes later, they already walked in and out. Bert had moved the chopping block in front of the window, so that the cats didn't have to jump too deep and that they were also able to get back into the kitchen again. Satisfied with his work, he rubbed his hands.

In the meantime, Kathrin had put all the dry food she could find in bowls and had placed them around the kitchen. She had also filled four pots with water and put them in different places. "That's it, pussycats. If you eat everything at once, you have to catch some mice," she said. Then she grinned. When Bert looked at her, wondering, she pointed to the bowls. "The best ones I could find, all of them Rosenthal. They shouldn't live like dogs, after all." Now Bert grinned as well.

Tom still looked grumpily. "Could you by any chance tell me why we didn't turn right way and leave last night?" Kathrin became serious. "If they were able to fool us like this, they should at least feel a little ashamed." And a little later she added, "Although they probably don't know what that means."

They were exhausted and satisfied but still a little shocked when they locked the door at about 7:00 a.m. They decided to put the key under the flowerpot next to the short stairs. "O.K., and now we go to the airport and take the next plane south," Bert announced. "Are you serious?" Kathrin looked dumbfounded. "Absolutely, honey, let's go." Tom looked at him admiringly.

"Man, you are really spontaneous. That's cool." And with that, they ran to the car, laughing.

"It's good to be home again," Kathrin said and raised her glass of wine to Bert. Tom had disappeared into his room and checked his e-mails. The three of them had a tan and looked relaxed. "We absolutely have to visit Turkey again," Bert remarked. "At least people there respect me as the head of the family." He grinned mischievously at his wife. She ran her fingers through her bleached hair and grinned back. "That's OK with me. And meanwhile I enjoy being wooed by the locals." "No you don't!" laughed Bert and kissed her.

The phone rang. Still laughing, Kathrin picked up the receiver. Then, her smile suddenly disappeared and the corners of her mouth sank; she looked almost grim. "Really? Hmm." Her voice sounded cold. Bert looked at her inquiringly. "Klaus!" she formed with her lips and he could almost see the exclamation mark. He was outraged and wanted to take the receiver away from her. That this idiot dared to call…. Instead, Kathrin put him on speakerphone.

Her eyes became bigger and bigger. "… We barely noticed that you were in our house. Really, everything was exactly the way we left it. How did you do that?" Klaus asked cheerfully at the other end. Kathrin was obviously at a loss for words. "But…that is…." Before she could continue, Klaus interrupted her again. "Just imagine what happened around here. This place is always so quiet, nothing going on. Shortly after we returned, we saw the police directly across the street from our house where old Mr. Mahlich used to live. You haven't seen him by any chance, have you? Well, you probably couldn't. The police said that he has been lying in his basement for at least two weeks. Dead. Probably drank himself to death. Yuck, that must have been a terrible smell. Maybe that was even planned. You know, he always seemed so sloppy. And, honestly, nobody around here thought that he would get very old. But imagine, before he died he must have cleaned the house thoroughly. Everything was sparkly clean except for a little bit of dust, says Udo. Udo works with the police, you know. So, and he put all the cat food out for his animals. And water too; that wasn't even spoilt. He even thought of the windows, so that the cats could get out." At this point he paused for a moment. Before Kathrin could cut in, he rattled on. " By the way, we have two cats now and the neighbours took another two. Sorry that I am telling you all this stuff. I just thought you might be interested. He must have been dead already by the time you stayed at our place. Disgusting, isn't it? The thought that there is a dead body just across the street! But the reason I am calling… Could you send us back the keys? We have some friends who would like to visit here next week. They would need the ke…" Kathrin put down the receiver very quietly. Then she sneezed explosively.

Conflict and Resolution

Kathrin suffered a stink conflict when she found out that her nice hosts didn't feel it was necessary to tidy up their house. Already during the cleaning she entered a hanging solution; she sneezed and she suddenly developed a running nose.

She also contracted a so-called allergy. Allergies are nothing but warnings of the body against a situation during which an individual was once hit by a severe DHS.

In the moment of the DHS, every detail of the surrounding circumstances gets registered as though it was captured on film. Colours, smells, voices, certain plants, and even the weather are burned into the biological memory.

Whenever one of these signals occurs, for example, the smell of the cleaner or the sight of a cat, the body immediately warns against it. It realizes very quickly that it was false alarm and moves from the short conflict active phase to the healing phase, which, depending on the individual case, manifests itself in a running nose, shortness of breath, runny eyes, etc.

Usually, people talk about an allergic cold or, in Kathrin's case, a doctor will presumably diagnose a cat allergy, because in the future her body will react with these symptoms to cats and their hair – if she doesn't manage to resolve the conflict internally.

The Kidnapping - or: The Catnapping
• Tapsy and the conjunctiva

"Tapsy hasn't come back yet." Thomas seemed worried. Nervously he looked at his watch. Automatically, Claudia did the same. "Since when is she been outside?" Thomas thought for a moment. "1:00 p.m. I haven't seen her since." That was four hours ago and very worrisome indeed. The little black cat, Tapsy, never stayed away for longer than an hour without stopping by in between. If she didn't show up for four hours, something happened to her. They looked at each other in a concerned manner. "I guess we will have to wait for a little while," said Thomas and sighed.

Tapsy hid under the couch. She didn't want to have anything to do with that girl. First, she seemed to be nice and Tapsy had let the girl pet her. But then, the strange girl had picked her up and Tapsy didn't like that at all. And before she was able to show her claws, the girl had put her in the backpack. "You will come with me. You'll see we will become friends."

At home the girl had taken Tapsy out of the backpack and quickly let her go when she showed her sharp claws. "Hey, stop that," the girl scolded her and sucked the scratch at her forearm. She glared at Tapsy who hid under the couch. The girl calmed down again. "You know what, I'll call you Blacky." From a distance, she looked at the collar with the phone number and the name. "And we will take off that thing as soon as we get along better." "Karla, lunch is ready," a voice called from outside. Quickly, the girl put her finger on her mouth. "You are quiet. Don't you dare to give us away." Then she left the room.

Tapsy had a look around. The room wasn't very big, but it had a few nice hiding places. Intrigued, she sniffed at a wadded shirt lying in one corner. After thinking about it for a minute, she stood on it with legs apart and peed on it. Then she cleaned herself and had another look around. She didn't find any food, but at least she could hide under the bed for now.

Thomas and Claudia were depressed. The children, as well, hung about quietly. Tapsy hadn't been home for two days now. "I don't think something bad happened to her," Claudia comforted Thomas. Tapsy was his favourite. I think she's all right. Maybe someone took her home." Thomas sighed. "Actually, I don't have such a bad feeling either," he agreed. I will make a few posters the boys can distribute. Maybe someone will call," said Claudia.

Tapsy just didn't get the opportunity to slip out of the door. She'd had enough. This strange girl wanted to pet her, but Tapsy had been able to avoid that so far, particularly because the girl was obviously afraid that her parents would find Tapsy. It was already the second day that the girl had given her some milk and dry food, but Tapsy was thirsty. Then she was lucky. Karla had watered her plants too much. Contentedly, Tapsy licked the water from the coaster. Then she did her business in the flowerpot. She deliberately ignored the makeshift litter box made from a shoebox.

Tapsy had been gone for four days. The family's spirits were down. Claudia had even put an ad in the paper. But it would only come out on Saturday; until then, the posters would have to do the job. Even the neighbours had inquired about Tapsy. Everyone liked the cat that was a little on the small side. She always looked particularly young and helpless, but she could be a very cruel hunter. The other cats missed her too. They all seemed anxious.

"You dirty little animal, you peed in my bed." Karla yelled angrily at Tapsy who hid in the corner. "Just wait." Furiously, she threw a show at the cat. "What is going on here?" Karla's mother stood in the door. Karla stared at her. Blacky had disappeared. Good. So, her mother didn't see her. "Uhm, nothing, mom, I am just practicing for our new play." Her mother looked at her suspiciously. "Can you keep it down a little? It sounds truly awful." With that, she left the room.

Tapsy had to find a way to escape. She wanted to leave. She wanted to go home. She wanted to have Thomas and Claudia back and she would never let any stranger pet her again. Unhappily, she sat at the window and stared outside. There wasn't a possibility anywhere. Even if the window had been open, it was too high. She would have hurt herself.

Would you like to have a little black cat from our litter? It looks exactly the way you described your cat." The caller virtually exuded a pushy cheerfulness. "No, thank you," Thomas said and tried to remain polite. "We want only our Tapsy back, not just any cat. Otherwise there are really enough other cats in the neighbourhood. He was exasperated when he hung up. All day long people had been calling; nobody had a tip so far, everyone just wanted to talk him into taking some cat. Tapsy hadn't turned up at the animal shelter either and, gradually, he was giving up hope.

Karla's father was reading the newspaper. As always, he skimmed through the classified section. "That's the last thing I would do. Just because of a cat," he growled hoarsely. "Pardon me?" Karla's mother seemed a little absent-minded. "I didn't hear you, darling." "That's the last thing I would do, to put an ad in the paper just because of a cat. These people are completely crazy." Then he threw the newspaper aside, took the remote control, and turned on a soccer game.

Karla had taken the newspaper to her room. "They are talking about you," she said discontentedly. "What a bummer. If my parents find out about that, I'll be in trouble." She looked at the cat and thought for a moment. "I have to get you out of here," she concluded. Then, she fetched her backpack. Just as she was trying to make the cat go into the backpack, the door opened and Karla's father grumbled, "Where is the paper?" Then he spotted Tapsy. Even before he could say anything, Tapsy scooted into the hallway and scurried into the next corner. At that moment the doorbell rang, and when Karla's mother opened the door, Tapsy ran out of the apartment like lightning and she didn't look back. She was lucky. The front door was open as well.

The sixth day. A Sunday. Claudia and Thomas avoided the topic of Tapsy. Since the morning they had been talking about this and that, but not about the cat. Claudia didn't even say anything when she discovered fresh paw prints at the balcony door. She had cleaned it only the other day. "Where did they come from?" she wondered. Maybe they were from another cat. On the other hand – only Tapsy used to stand in front of the window pane scratching to let them know that she wanted to go out or come inside. Shaking her head, she went to the kitchen to make coffee.

The four of them were sitting at the table. Breakfast was silent. Claudia felt she was being watched. Lost in thought she turned her head to the balcony door. Her eyes became big. In front of the door there was Tapsy.

Tired and exhausted, Tapsy had curled up in Thomas's bedspread. Finally she was home again. After an exciting welcome they had cuddled and spoilt her. First, Tapsy had to check whether things were OK everywhere around the house, but now she was really exhausted.

"O, you poor thing." Thomas petted Tapsy. She purred; then a sneeze shook the small furry body again and again. She looked at him with cloudy eyes. Her right eye was inflamed. The conjunctiva constantly secreted some puss. Thomas carefully removed the accumulation from the corner of her eye. Tapsy let it happen. "If her condition doesn't improve, we have to take her to the vet," Claudia worried. "Just wait a little. I think it is getting better already."

He was right. A few days later Tapsy felt better again. The cold was gone and her eye was clear again. The boys had collected the posters and all the neighbours had inquired about her condition. Claudia watched how Tapsy was on her way to walking along the sidewalk. A couple walked towards her. "O, you are so pretty," the woman said enthusiastically and bent down to Tapsy. Obviously, she wanted to pet her. Like a shot, Tapsy turned around, ran a few meters back and quickly climbed the wire netting fence. She jumped into her own garden where she watched the couple from a safe distance while she was cleaning herself. A little disappointed the woman gazed after her. "But I didn't want to harm you."

Conflict and Resolution

What applies for humans, applies also for other mammals. Tapsy had suffered a stink conflict and, in addition, a visual separation conflict when she lost sight of Thomas, with whom she has a special connection.

As she is right-pawed and considers Thomas an equal partner, she suffered the conflict on the partner side. During the healing phase she contracted a massive cold and conjunctivitis.

Note: The biological laws of the New Medicine apply not only to humans.

Not Without My Daughter

• Gerd and the bronchitis

"No, that is not possible. You can't do that. Carolin isn't able to care for our daughter. She is too immature. Please, don't do that." Gerd almost pleaded. But it was in vain. "Every mother is better than the best father." With these words the judge introduced his verdict. With these words Gerd lost his daughter. Paula had to stay with Carolin.

"Just wait, son, it may not get as bad as you think." His mother tried to comfort Gerd, but her comfort seemed empty. She, too, knew what Paula had to go through now. Carolin would make life difficult for her daughter. But what could they do? The law had decided in favour of the mother. And it had disregarded the reality of the situation.

Up to that point, Gerd had raised his daughter by himself. Shortly after the birth, Carolin came to him and said, "Here, you care for her, you are the father." With that, she had handed him a half-year-old baby and a backpack before she turned and left. He hadn't seen her in a year until she suddenly returned. And, of course, she wanted Paula back.

"She is like a child who wants to have its toy back," Gerd had told the judge. "But our daughter isn't a toy. She is a human being. And her home is now with me. She doesn't know her mother any more." That hadn't changed anything. The judge granted Carolin sole custody. He wasn't even granted access. After all, they weren't married.

The following weeks went by like in a bad dream, a nightmare. After work, he often walked by the house Carolin and Paula lived in. He always hoped to get a quick look at his daughter. One time, it almost took his breath away when he saw a woman with a stroller. When she turned around, he realized that it wasn't Carolin.
It was the fourth time that the phone rang. Obtrusive. Up to then, Gerd simply hadn't picked up. But, gradually, the constant ringing became annoying. He picked up. "Yes," he answered impatiently. "Hey, you are the guy the kid, Paula, belongs to, right?" The voice at the other end babbled. Immediately, Gerd was alerted. "What happened to her," he demanded. "Well, you know, she has already been with us for three days and her stupid mother won't show up." "What?" Gerd's thoughts were racing. "Where do I find you?" He forced himself to ask calmly. "Go to 6 Karlsplatz; the name is Bause. That's me. But hurry, the bawling is annoying."

Gerd hasted in record speed to the Karlsplatz, which was just around the corner. He arrived there out of breath, rang the doorbell, and almost ran over a sleazy guy who had remained standing in the doorway. The apartment looked as if a bomb had hit it with garbage and clutter including leftover food, beer bottles, and clothes. Then he saw his daughter. Paula was sitting in the corner, her face covered in tears. He could see the trace of a hand on her cheek and she had her fingers in her mouth. Gerd approached her. When she saw him she started smiling. "Dad," she said. Then she babbled things he couldn't understand.

"Where did she learn that?" Gerd asked himself. After all, she hadn't seen him in a while, and at the time he lost the lawsuit, she hadn't started talking, although she was about to. He quickly dropped the thought. Carrying Paula, he turned to the drunken man. "You hit her. Do you want to hit me too, or do you just hit babies?" His anger grew. The man held his arms in front of his face to protect himself. "Hey, man, that wasn't me. Carolin did that. Before she took off, she slapped the kid because it wouldn't shut up. And since then she is gone."

"Did she call? Did she say what she wanted to do?" Still angry, Gerd glared at the man. But he had calmed down a little. The man seemed to have noticed the change. Absent-mindedly he grabbed a bottle of beer and opened it. After he had had a gulp, he wiped with his hands across his mouth. "She didn't say anything. Just that she'd had enough. I found your number in the kid's backpack. Otherwise I would have called the police." He nodded and then he slumped into a shabby armchair. "Take her and go. There is her backpack. He pointed to the couch before he had another gulp from the bottle.

As fast as possible Gerd ran home with Paula. Hopefully, nobody would notice the dirty clothes the girl was wearing. It would have embarrassed him. After they came home, he gave her a bath and dressed her in clean clothes. He had already bought them a few months ago, but they had been too big at that time. Then he thought about the next steps that had to be undertaken.

"It's not that easy because you are not married. For now, child services will keep an eye on her before a decision will be made in regards to where the child will stay." Gerd looked at the woman in disbelief. "Excuse me? You want to give the child back to the mother who so badly neglected her?" The woman shook her head. "That is also a possibility, but it seems unlikely at the moment. Apart from that, we consider a children's home or foster care. After all, there is a court decision denying you custody."

Gerd just stared at the woman. Then he mumbled angrily between his lips, "You can be certain that I won't have Paula taken away from me again. Just try it." "Well, Mr. Renner, if you force us to, we will certainly take the necessary steps. The case is neither in your nor in our hands. There are laws, you know." She got up, gave him her business card, and walked towards the door. "We will contact you regarding the further procedure."

Again, Gerd felt like being in a nightmare. Carolin hadn't shown up again since her disappearance. Some of her friends claimed that she had left for South America. Gerd didn't care. She could stay wherever she wanted as long as it was far away from him and Paula. During these weeks, his daughter was his only comfort. Only now he realized how much he had missed her. They enjoyed every minute together. She chuckled when she saw him and she could already talk in whole sentences. He was fascinated by his daughter. But in the background was this constant fear of the possibility that they would take her away again.

".... It is the court's decision that the father is granted full custody. The mother's address is unknown...." Gerd didn't hear the rest of it. He felt incredibly happy and relieved when the judge spoke those words. Again, a lawsuit had been necessary, because child services wanted to take Paula away from him and put her in foster care. But he didn't let them take her. When they arrived with the police, he already had a temporary injunction in his hands. The childcare workers looked a little sheepishly when they left. One of the police officers had given him a friendly nod. That had been four weeks ago. Now the court had decided in his favour. He still couldn't believe his luck.

Gerd lay awake. The persistent cough prevented him from falling asleep. It had been like this for days and his condition didn't seem to improve. The doctor had diagnosed bronchitis and had prescribed all kinds of drugs. When he read about the side effects, he did without most of them. He tried not to cough too hard, because he didn't want to wake up Paula. Although he was on sick leave, he didn't get much sleep. During the nights, he was lying awake most of the time and fell asleep only in the early morning hours. But then, it wasn't long before Paula woke him up with her babbling and talking. Though he was very tired and his chest hurt, he enjoyed her presence. His cough would go away, but Paula would stay with him; he was certain about that.

Conflict and Resolution

Gerd has suffered a conflict of threat to the territory when the court granted custody to the mother and he lost his daughter. Later, when he had gotten back his daughter but child services threatened to put her in a children's home, he was set on the track.

During a conflict of threat to the territory the individual experiences fear for his or her territory – his or her house, the car, or the apartment – or for the content of the territory. That could be the family, the children, or the pet. The conflict is always with a certain person or office, e.g., the tax office, the police, or an organization. Gerd was afraid that Paula would be taken away from him again. He developed an ulcer in the bronchial mucosa.

When the court granted him custody, the conflict was resolved and a swelling of the epithelial tissue occurred, which resulted in a lack of ventilation. The consequence was the bad cough; bronchitis was diagnosed. Often, such a cough can last for months and cause serious pain.

Lord Porn
• Peter and the large intestine

"You are put on leave. Right now, I don't have a choice. You have to understand. First, I need to have the case investigated." The director shook Peter Keller's hand briefly, pulled it back quickly, and said goodbye. Peter Keller was stunned. His thoughts were racing again and again around this one point: put on leave. He was put on leave.

Peter Keller was considered to be the most diligent accountant the company ever had. Being 46 years old, he was considerably younger than he looked. He seemed a little dusty, a boring guy with thin hair who was always wearing the same grey suits. His coworkers assumed that he had to have at least twelve of them.

For 25 years, Keller had been working for the company. Always reliable, he never missed a day. Even on days he didn't feel that well he had shown up for work. And why not? He didn't have a wife or a family. Peter Keller lived for his job. And now this.

Overnight they had kicked him out because of unproven allegations and suspicions. His computer had been the deciding factor. Already fifteen years ago when the computers had been introduced, he had had the feeling that he wouldn't necessarily make friends with that technology. Finally, he had come to terms with it though. Ten years ago, when they all got Internet access, he didn't care. He hardly ever used it. He found the things he needed to know in his reference books on the shelf.

But now his world had fallen apart. And it was the fault of the Internet. It all started with a search. Suddenly the police appeared and had boxed and taken all the computers. There protest was in vain. The officers acted by order of the district attorney's office. "Suspicion of child pornography," one officer had told them laconically. And shortly after, the whole department had been without equipment.

The boss had sent them home. The following day, replacement computers had been installed. Working with the unfamiliar device was strange. But, after all, Peter Keller was able to work again. And that's what he did. Until now. Now he was put on leave.

He walked slowly down the hallway; he barely noticed the glances of his colleagues, or their whispering. "I always thought that something is wrong with him...no family...somehow twisted..." They had remained strangers to him. Peter Keller didn't have friends. But up until then he believed that he wouldn't have enemies either. Obviously, he was wrong. Somebody had played a dirty trick on him.

"How did these pictures and videos get on your computer?" The same question for the tenth time. Peter Keller helplessly shrugged his shoulders. "I don't know. Really. I don't watch something like that. I work with the computer. I am almost never on the Internet. I don't have an explanation."

"Well, well," said the investigator who was in his thirties. "Never on the Internet? We checked that. Your computer has its own IP-address within the company network. And that address is almost constantly online." He pushed a pile of paper over to Peter. They were protocols about Internet sessions apparently emanating from his computer with his IP-address. Peter Keller shook his head in disbelief. "That is impossible, seriously, you have to believe me." And how do you think did that happen?" the investigator asked and sat on the edge of the table. "You surely must have a password, right?" Keller literally collapsed. "Of course I do. No one except me has access to the computer."

Keller was standing at the window. For hours he had been watching the street. What else could he do anyway? It was raining. Nobody was waiting for him. He was still put on leave. For two months already. They couldn't fire him until they had evidence that he was guilty. But the police still investigated. Thinking of the accusations sent chills up and down his spine. They had found thousands of data with child pornography on his computer, obviously well hidden. He couldn't explain how they had gotten there. Apparently, nobody believed that he despised something like that. That he would never dream of looking at such twisted stuff. Peter Keller was at a loss. He couldn't believe that his colleagues contemplated him as being a bad guy.

Recently, he had also developed some health problems. Sometimes he experienced a bit of a dragging pain in the lower abdomen, which he didn't consider very serious. But he suffered from indigestion. He had tried everything from laxatives to sports, but nothing worked. Somehow it was a problem. It didn't hurt; well, sometimes a little bit but mostly it didn't. He didn't want to go to the doctor. If it was serious, it was supposed to be that way. It wasn't important any longer anyway.

The phone rang. It was an unusual sound for Peter Keller. He picked up the receiver, "Hello?" "Hello, Mr. Keller. I am calling to notify you of a positive development. Evidently, the police found the child pornography dealer who used your computer. You are exonerated. Yesterday they made an arrest in the company. I would be happy if you would come back to work, now, that all the misunderstandings have been cleared up." The voice of his boss seemed almost sleazy. Keller clenched inside. His hand touched his belly. "I have to do something." The thought suddenly flashed into his mind. "I see. And who has been arrested?" he asked. "Schreiber, our system administrator. Just imagine. He obviously used your computer because you are hardly ever online and are not interested in computers. That's why you didn't realize what was going on." Keller hung up slowly.

Schreiber had misused Keller's computer for months. That's what the investigator had explained to him later, when he made the effort and visited him at home. "I have to apologize," he said and he added, "I knew from the beginning that you weren't guilty. You didn't know enough about computers to hide the data that cleverly. And you would have covered your tracks much better. But we had to let everybody go on believing that you are guilty in order to find the real criminal." Keller had listened to him and had nodded. He didn't bother to comment. Meanwhile, he had other problems. His intestine didn't function any more.

Everybody had greeted him more or less friendly. Many of his colleagues seemed to have a guilty conscience and assured him that they hadn't doubted his innocence in the first place. Keller watched them silently; he didn't talk much. These colleagues would never be more than strangers to him. And that was the nicest thing that crossed his mind when he thought about them. He started clearing the work that had piled up on his desk.

In hindsight, the story of the twisted system administrator wasn't nearly as exciting. Schreiber had used Keller's computer via remote control. He had had every password and every access. Using swap markets, he downloaded the pictures and videos, burned them on CDs and sold them. Nobody would have ever found out about if it hadn't been for an investigator who picked up Schreiber's track at the swap market. The cover of another twelve suspects had been blown, however, not from their company.

Peter Keller worked like he always did. After this experience he had even less contact with his colleagues. Sometimes he had the feeling his boss would have preferred to get rid of him. But all these observations were just marginally. He had other problems. For several days now he was having bloody stools. Sometimes it was so severe that he had considered going to the doctor. But then he dismissed the possibility. How would seeing a doctor help him? If that's how it was meant to be, that's how it would be. He would just continue doing his job.

Absent-mindedly, Peter Keller was standing at his desk. He felt his lower abdomen, but it didn't hurt. He continued to have bloody stools, but he was glad that, at least, it was working again. It didn't matter whether it was bloody or not. Actually, he felt much better. Relieved. Then a smile went over his face. "If that's how it is meant to be, that's how it will be." With this thought on his mind he sat down at his desk, turned on the computer, and wrote his notice.

Conflict and Resolution

Peter Keller suffered a classic conflict of nasty, indigestible anger. He, who was always reliable and decent, was suddenly suspected of having downloaded child pornography from the Internet. If that wasn't enough, they simply put him, who had been a reliable employee for many years, on leave.

During the conflict active phase, he developed a cauliflower-like adenocarcinoma in the large intestine. It grew and relocated the intestine, so that it was a problem for his stools to go through. The problem lasted up to the point where Keller's conflict was resolved, which happened when the person who was the true criminal, was found. From that moment on, the decomposition of the tumor through bacteria or tuberculosis began and it resulted in bloody stools.

A nasty, mean shit conflict can also cause colorectal cancer. During a nasty, mean shit conflict, the cancer develops in the upper rectum.

The dangerous thing about colorectal cancer is always an impending intestinal obstruction. In that case, the patient needs surgery. However, it is sufficient to remove the tumor; other tissue doesn't have to be removed. As soon as there is bloody stool, the healing phase has started. From this moment on the risk of an intestinal obstruction occurring is only minimal unless it is a hanging resolution, in which case the risk still exists.

Victim of Insider Relationships
• Tom and the lumbago

He felt really good about it. Whistling inside, he left the room and thought about the conversation again. Yes, he was sure he would get the job, his dream job. While he put on his coat, Tom looked around the room contentedly. There was a young woman in her mid-twenties, pretty, blond hair, and slim figure.

He nodded to her and she smiled back. "Don't worry, the people are very nice," he said, because he believed to have detected a little bit of insecurity on her part. "O, did you apply as well?" she asked. Tom nodded and examined her. Suddenly he had a strange feeling. Worry? But why? It was impossible that this kid should be his competition. The woman looked as if she had just finished university. No chance compared to his experience. Again, he nodded to her and said goodbye.

Five days later, Tom held his portfolio in his hands. He tried to understand what was written there. "....We have to inform you...decided in favour of another applicant...with equal qualification...best success..." He couldn't believe it. He had never been so wrong about something.

He fell into his chair and stared at the letter. Should his feelings have so completely deceived him? The dream of the dream job was over. He would continue to hang out in the administration of the municipal office, be annoyed with boring routine, and probably get laid off soon due to whatever internal reasons.

Tom stared at his feet. He was still dumbfounded. "Don't worry about it, honey. It is their loss!" His wife approached him and gave him a kiss. He looked at her absent-mindedly. "Right," he just replied. Then he got up. He couldn't talk to her about it right now. He felt like blocked. He didn't want to either. He had to go to work.

His feelings hadn't deceived him. The blond, young woman had got his job. The question who had beaten him had bothered him ever since. So he had made some inconspicuous inquiries. As a matter of fact, she had his job now. And, as a matter of fact, he had been right from the beginning. She had just finished university, had no experience and hadn't published anything yet. It was a mystery to him why she had gotten this job.

Maybe someone had thought with his lower extremities. There was hardly another explanation. But that didn't comfort him. It hit him harder than he wanted to admit. Did being 40 years of age make him already too old? Would he ever be able to do something that he really liked and that would keep his family afloat? He didn't know. But he was deeply depressed.

He would have liked to talk with somebody about it. Not with his wife, though. She would just worry even more, which wasn't of any help to him. And his best friend, Mike, was on vacation. He was on a fishing trip in Norway. Tom sighed and grit his teeth. He could deal with it himself.

Great. Now, that he had finally overcome the anger about the muffed application according to the motto "Who knows what it is good for" he had to get sick on top of everything. He had a sore throat and he could barely swallow. Wearily, he walked to the bathroom and, with a small flashlight, had a look at his throat. His tonsils were deep red with little yellow specks. "Shoot," he thought.

From previous experience, Tom knew that a strep tonsillitis would knock him out completely. Nothing made him as sick as a tonsillitis. He would just be able to make it to the doctor to get a sick note. Then he had a week of suffering in front of him.

Whistling cheerfully, Tom entered his office. He was feeling well and recovered. "Good morning," he called out to his colleagues and walked over to his office. His secretary had put a list of appointments on his desk.

He scanned through the papers, paused for a minute, and wrinkled his forehead. "Looks like I will officially meet my little competition today," he mumbled to himself. "Did you say something, Mr. Bohm?" asked his secretary and looked at him. "No, no, Mrs. Kepler, nothing of importance. Can you tell me what this appointment is about?" He pointed with his finger to the sheet of paper. "The man was a little vague. As far as I understood, they need a building permit for a laboratory. He wanted to discuss the details with you." "The man? Are you sure? I thought that a woman is the head of the department." Tom frowned. "No, no. I am sure it is a man," his secretary insisted. Thoughtfully, Tom put the paper aside.

It turned out to be an interesting day. Tom's secretary had been right. Instead of the young, blond woman, a man appeared who was about Tom's age. He looked bland, presented his issue, and only discussed what was absolutely necessary. Eventually, Tom managed to bring him out of his shell; the guy was crazy about fishing. Tom didn't know anything about that topic, however, he learned a little bit from his friend Mike. It was enough for Edwin Kammer, who became more and more talkative.

Carefully, Tom directed the conversation towards Kammer's job. "I have this job since February. It is really not bad. You know, actually I was supposed to start already in January. The position had to be filled by then, otherwise it would have been cancelled. But I couldn't come to an agreement with my former employer," he gave away.

"I really began to worry that it wouldn't work out, but somehow my boss managed to keep the job for me. He grinned complacently and touched his belly. "Between you and me, we knew each other for quite a while and you just make certain things happen." He leaned back, looked at his watch, and got up. "I almost lost track of the time. So, it would be nice if we could sort this out quickly. I will be in contact with you again next week." Kammer reached out his hand to Tom. Tom took it, unmoved on the surface, but inside he was disgusted.

He breathed a sigh of relief after Kammer had left. After three phone calls he knew the whole story and he could have explained to this jerk exactly how his boss had managed to keep the position open for him. He had hired the young woman to fill the job and a month later, during the probation period, he had fired her again without giving any reasons. Instead, Edwin Kammer, the candidate they had already decided on long ago, started the job the inexperienced graduate, who was probably devastated, had to leave shortly before. "These jerks," Tom thought and shook his head. It was a good thing he didn't get that job. He was glad he didn't have to work with people like that.

That evening, he told his wife everything. Kathrin was used to quite a bit; she was working in a private company. But this affected her. "Just imagine how this young woman must have felt. Such a failure right at the beginning of her career!"

She was appalled when she looked at her husband and said, "They knew they wouldn't be able to treat you like that. They realized that you are not suited at all to become their victim. Now you know why you didn't have a chance." Tom nodded. Kathrin was right. It hadn't appeared to him until now. He wouldn't have let them get away with that kind of behaviour quite so easily.

"You know what," he said and kissed his wife, "let us go out and have a glass of wine. He got up and pulled her up as well. She laughed and kissed him back. "Exactly, let's celebrate because we were lucky and got away." She grinned and sprinted to the bathroom.

"Ouch, ah, ah, what the heck is this?" Startled, his secretary looked in the door. Tom couldn't stand up straight and held his back with his right hand. With the left hand he leaned on the table. "Do you want me to get a doctor for you. I am sure that is lumbago. Sometimes, my husband also has lumbago. You poor thing." Sympathetically, she helped him sit down in his chair. Tom groaned with pain.

The pain was excruciating. "No, thanks. It has to go without. But more than likely I won't be able to sit." He tried to get up again from the chair, leaned on the windowsill and closed his eyes for a moment.

"You look very pale, Mr. Bohm. Wouldn't it be better to get a doctor?" But Tom refused. "Maybe you could get me a painkiller, so that I get through the meeting," he asked. "Of course," she said and while she was leaving, Tom sadly mumbled, "Apparently, I am getting old."

Conflict and Resolution

Tom suffered a DHS with two aspects. First, there is the conflict of "being unable to grasp the chunk": He was convinced that he would get the new job, until someone else snapped it up. Second, he suffered a collapse of his self-esteem when he found out that they had chosen an inexperienced, young woman instead of him.

During the conflict active phase, the tonsils were enlarged. When he came to terms with his failure – "Who knows what it is good for" – the conflict was resolved. Tom contracted a strep tonsillitis.

The collapse of his self-esteem caused cell death in the connective tissue of the groin area during the conflict active phase, which lasted several weeks. When he found out that the reason for the rejection wasn't lacking qualification, but, on the contrary, they considered him too smart for their games, the conflict was resolved. Several days later, Tom had lumbago.

More severe cases show the development of edemas in the vertebrae areas during the healing phase, which leads to the intervertebral disks pushing through at the lumbar spine. While the healing advances, the size goes back to normal and everything slides back into place.

Law and Justice
• Hagen and the tinnitus

"Previously convicted! Now you are previously convicted," it pounded in Hagen's head. The same words over and over again. He realized that he was almost in some kind of a shock. Just now, the judge had found him guilty of assault. She had talked about disproportionate behaviour and the guy had grinned at him. Despite the fact that he was only 19, he gave the impression of being square-built. He sat in the audience; he obviously didn't want to miss this.

Sonny was the only child of a judge here at the local court of the small city. Hagen didn't know that when he pulled him away from the old woman and hit him with his fist first in the stomach and then on the chin. It wouldn't have mattered to him anyway.

The woman was about 70, small and delicate. She looked almost fragile and he saw the fear of death in her eyes. He couldn't help but step in. In a situation like this, he always had to think about his own grandmother who had also been small and delicate but resolute. Probably she would even have defended herself successfully against this guy; she had been very smart. "I still miss her," it went through his mind. That surprised him. He would have thought that the memory faded with the passing years, but it had become even more vivid instead.

"Twenty years? It has been that long?" He turned the numbers over in his mind. Right, it had been 20 years since the death of his grandmother. He had only been 13 at that time and it had pulled the rug out from under him. He had loved her very much.

Hagen would have helped anyone who was threatened. He simply had a very strong sense of justice. "Too strong," as his teachers had always said. They were often moved when Hagen stood up for fellow students because he thought they were being treated unfairly. It had brought him many enemies and only few thankyous. But that didn't matter to him. He couldn't help it.

At that particular evening, he only noticed the guy in the last moment. He was walking down the street absent-mindedly. His daughter wasn't feeling well. She had had pain in the knee for several days. He thought about what might have happened. Probably she had had problems during physical education. Lucie was only 8 years old, but she loved playing handball. And she just didn't like it when someone else was faster than her. She liked it best when she could run ahead, jump forward at the half circle and shoot the ball through the goaltender's legs. If somebody was faster than her, she had to work her way through the defense and didn't have a clear area to shoot. She hated that. "That's probably the reason," he had thought when, suddenly, he heard a hissing.

"Give it to me, old woman, or I'll kill you," a voice had snarled. Then, Hagen had heard a gasp. When he turned around, he looked directly in the old woman's eyes and saw that she was scared to death. Stubbornly, she held on to her handbag.
A tall guy stood in front of her, holding one strap of the bag and stroke out to hit her. Hagen didn't think for another minute. He jumped forward, pulled the

guy around and hit him with his fist on the solar plexus. In order to ensure that he was knocked out, Hagen added another right hook. The guy kissed the dust and didn't move any more.

That had happened two month ago. "Previously convicted," went through Hagen's mind again. The judge had sentenced him to half a year with probation. In addition, he had to pay a 1500 Euro fine. It rang in his ears in the truest sense of the word. He heard a buzzing and whistling noise in his left ear. It annoyed him and he shook his head, but the noises wouldn't disappear.

In the beginning, the judge was actually quite nice. She was in her early forties, athletic, short hair cut. "But corrupt," Hagen thought now and clenched his fist unconsciously. The attacker had just sustained a few bruises. But Hagen was convicted of assault.

"That is disproportionate, judge," he thought and shook his head. The youngster just got a few hours of community service, because he hadn't offended before and had to be treated according to the juvenile criminal law. That's what the explanatory statement of the same judge had said just a few weeks before.

Hagen didn't have any idea how they had managed it. Actually, it was robbery, but they had turned it into theft. A huge difference. In the former case the guy would have been sentenced to at least a year, while in the latter case the sentence started with paying a fine. And because he still went to school – "to high school of all things," Hagen thought and shook his head – he just had to work a few hours in a social institution.

Hagen remembered the guy's grinning. Then he remembered the face of the old woman. The mugging had left her speechless. She couldn't even scream. She just stood there, clung to her purse, and trembled.

"The fellow would have been surprised," Hagen thought. The woman had had neither money nor a credit card on her. The content of the purse was useless for the attacker. It contained just an old photo album. She had taken it home from her sister to keep it safe. She had told Hagen later that her sister was confused. The woman didn't want the memories to disappear. Family photos; the parents, the brother who had passed away a long time ago, and mutual friends. "I wouldn't have given it to him either," thought Hagen and his thoughts wandered back to Lucie. "My daughter won't have a father who is previously convicted," he decided. If necessary, he would have to go through all the instances. "But I am not just going to sit here and take that."

This decision made him feel better immediately. Determinedly, he lifted his head. And he saw fear of death. He knew that look. This time, he saw it on the face of a woman in her early forties, athletic, with a short haircut. Three guys had surrounded her and threatened her with a knife.

"Help me," she demanded. There was nothing left of the judge's former equanimity. "Why doesn't she take her BMW but walks instead," Hagen asked himself. At the same time, he felt this deep disgust again for the judge, but also for the attackers. They watched him from the corners of their eyes, assessing him and how dangerous he could be to them. Three guys, maybe

16 or 17 years old. Probably not the sons of judges, otherwise they had chosen a different victim.

"Keep out of this, old man," one of the three said and waved his knife. Hagen grinned. Then he walked towards them. The judge looked at him hopefully. "Can't you hear," griped a second, somewhat heavier, guy. "Listen, boys," Hagen started, "You are committing a robbery here. You will get at least a year behind bars, unless daddy is a judge or something similar. Well, is he?" Hagen asked and looked at the three guys. They had a confused expression on their faces. One of them shook his head. "Nope, unemployed," he said almost automatically. His friends poked him in the ribs with their elbows. "Shut up, Chucki. That's none of his business," a tall blond guy grumbled. He stared at Hagen with narrow eyes. "What was that all about, old man? Do you want to get in trouble?" But this threat didn't sound very convincing.

Hagen shook his head. Then he approached them. "Robbery is really tricky. Maybe you should try theft. May I?" He took the briefcase from the judge who gave it to him unresistingly. He bowed. "Thank you." Then he turned around, put the briefcase down, and turned towards the trio again. "So, you are walking along the street, see the briefcase, and ask yourselves what might be in there." The three guys looked at him blankly. "Go ahead, have a look." The small fat one walked to the briefcase, opened it, and searched the content. "Hmm, some papers, a key, some photos, an apple, and a wallet," he mumbled to himself. Then he took the latter and looked at it more closely. "Hey, lots of money in here. All together, several thousand bucks for sure," he reported to his cronies enthusiastically.

"Well, actually, being the honest finders you are, you would have to turn it in, right?" The three of them stared at Hagen as though he was an alien. "Anything else, old man?" asked the third guy who had been quiet so far. "You are really crazy." "But everything else would be considered theft," Hagen explained. Then he looked at the trio. "How old are you anyway, 16?" The plump one nodded before the tall guy could prevent it. "Then you won't have any problems. For having committed a theft, you just have to pay a small fine, or, in your case, a few hours of community service if you get caught. Not like robbery, where they put you in prison together with murderers." Hagen continued, "But I have a better idea."

"We don't see honest guys like you around here very often. Most of them steal the handbags of old ladies," said the officer at the station while he let the judge confirm the receipt of her briefcase. "But you must know that better than I do," he added and grinned her. "Pretty big sum of money you are carrying around, hey? 10,000 Euros. What would you need all that cash for? He asked curiously. She looked uncomfortable. "Sometimes you just need it." She squeezed the words out curtly. "Our boys here will be happy about the reward; ten per cent isn't bad, after all." Jovially, he folded his hands across his belly and looked to the side where three 16-year-old boys were standing. They appeared insecure. Repeatedly, they forced themselves to smile, because a photographer constantly took their photos. A real storm of flashlights was unleashed at the station while the officer kept asking them questions: Where did they find the briefcase, why hadn't they just kept it, whether all that money wasn't the least bit tempting. By looking at the boys it was obvious that they were overwhelmed.

With a pinched expression on her face, the judge looked at the boys as well. She thought about something, and made a decision. She was just about to say something when a police officer turned towards her again. "I thought that the press should report about this case, because it doesn't happen very often. That's why I called and they sent the photographer. I am sure you won't mind a little publicity. It will certainly serve as a good example." He grinned like the cat that licked the cream.

The next morning, Hagen studied the newspaper. He grinned when he saw the headline and the photo in the local section. It showed a woman with a short hair and an athletic figure in her early forties. She presented several banknotes to three teenagers, who appeared to be quite insecure. The smile on her face seemed a little forced. The caption read: "Judge thanks honest finders with 1000 Euros. 'Honesty deserves to be rewarded', she said." Absent-mindedly, Hagen touched his ear. He had the feeling it was getting worse. But that couldn't spoil his good mood.

Still grinning, Hagen picked up the receiver, dialed the number of the police station, and waited. He was lucky. His cousin answered the phone immediately. "Well done, Ingo, I owe you."

Conflict and Resolution

Hagen suffered a so-called hearing conflict during this situation, which he perceived as "unreal". It is one of the many biological conflicts that often unconsciously determine our everyday life and that nature created as a protection program. In this case, the conflict content is: I couldn't believe my ears; I couldn't believe what I just heard." That's what happened to Hagen when the judge found him guilty, which came as a complete surprise to him. From that moment on, he was hearing buzzing and whistling in his left ear, called tinnitus.

Indeed, these very uncomfortable ear noises have a biological function. They are the expression of the suffered and active hearing conflict. The noises and sounds represent signal sounds and function as a warning, that is, a warning of a danger connected to the acoustical information. In Hagen's case, the judge's words during the proclamation of the sentence were the trigger of his conflict. But she was also crucial for him entering the healing- or conflict resolved phase. At this point, in the case of tinnitus, the person involved suffers acute hearing loss; the hearing ability of the right ear is rapidly deteriorating. Naturally and inevitably, Hagen experienced these symptoms as well.

Once the healing phase is finished, the hearing ability is usually improving again, unless the person suffers so-called relapses, or conflict specific recurrences, during the healing phase. That means that the conflict active phase started immediately in the moment of the first conflict experience when the person was unable or didn't want to process the chunk of information he or she heard, as was the case with Hagen. Simultaneously, our brain also stores the circumstances and perceptions accompanying this negative experience just like a snapshot.

The resolution of a hearing conflict can result in lasting hardness of hearing or even deafness.

The Surprise

• Marie and the larynx

Marie's hands trembled while she was turning over the pages of the photo album. She saw the pictures of her mother, her father, and her brother. It had been such a long time ago. Now she was 70 and almost alone. Only her sister was still alive. But in a different time: She suffered from Alzheimer's.

Marie had to think constantly of that evening when this man had mugged her. He was still almost a child. But she had seen his eyes. There was nothing but indifference and coldness. "He would have stabbed me," she recollected. She recognized a murderer when she saw one. During the last days of the war there had been many of his kind around. They were Germans and Russians, always just a few among many. But that had been enough. One of them had put her uncle up against the wall. "You fascist," he had yelled. He didn't have that indifference in his eyes, only madness and death. He had pulled the trigger of his Kalashnikov and had virtually riddled his uncle with bullets. Her mother had been stunned. "Me, too," she remembered. They had tried in vain to convince the Russian soldier that her uncle was harmless. As long as she could think he had been like a child. The other people in the village had called him retarded. It had been very difficult and needed some tricks to save him from the Nazis' euthanasia program, only for the Russian to shoot him.

Thoughtfully, Marie turned over another page. At that time she had gotten to know the eyes of the murderers. Not all of them had been like that Russian. Many of them were nice in the beginning, but soon showed their true faces. A German officer had been like that. She remembered that as well. He was on the run when he came to the village and mobilized the *Volkssturm*. They were boys and fragile old men who were supposed to defend the bridge against the approaching Russian soldiers. Her mother didn't want to let her brother go. "He is only 13 years old," she had screamed and stepped in front of Jürgen. "Old enough," the officer had barked and pushed her aside. Then, he had given the delicate boy, who was too small for his age, a gun and had sent him to join the others.

Jürgen miraculously survived. Her mother had been overjoyed. Up until the day when her uncle was killed. After that, she completely changed. She rarely talked and was absent-minded. She only went back to being herself after she had saved the women of the village from being raped. At that time, Marie hadn't understood what her mother did. Now, in hindsight, she admired her quick wit and her courage. A dozen completely drunken men had come to the village. They had had some kind of celebration. And then they knocked at the front doors of the houses. First with their fists and, later, they kicked the doors with their feet. They bellowed in a foreign language. The houses were all overcrowded at that time. There was no building where families of refugees and the owners hadn't been cooped up in.

Marie remembered as if it was yesterday how her mother got up, got dressed, put on her coat, and ran outside. She was terribly worried about her. "Go away, go away, njet," she shouted over and over again and ran towards the Russians, her hands waving. First the soldiers glared at her blankly; then they staggered towards her. "Njet, everybody is sick. Everybody has diphtheria," she yelled. That was a word the soldiers knew. They seemed to sober up instantly. Uncertainly, they looked at each other, then at the house, and to her mother. "Eta prawda?" one of them asked suspiciously. "Prawda, prawda," her mother confirmed quickly.

The soldiers didn't check whether she had really told them the truth. They turned around, grumbling. They also didn't touch her mother. When she walked a step towards them, they almost stumbled while trying to get away from her. "Dawai, domoi," was the watchword, and then they retreated.

Marie sighed and put the photo album aside. "I wonder whether this boy is actually aware of the harm he nearly caused." That album contained the only memories of her family she had left. If she had lost it…. She didn't even dare to think about that possibility. Ironically, she had decided that very day that the album wasn't safe enough with her sister any longer. "If it hadn't been for that nice man," she thought, shaking her head.

She still remembered very vividly the moment the robber stood in front of her, demanding her handbag. But she was lucky. Somehow, all of them had been lucky. Even during the war. In spite of all those terrible experiences they had survived; most of her family members, at any rate. They had been sick frequently. All of them had contracted tuberculosis soon after the war was really over, meaning that the Russians, as well, had left. After the murder of the uncle, her mother had experienced several signs of palsy and the doctor thought she might have suffered strokes. But the symptoms abated. Marie made some tea. She would say thank you to the man who rescued her. She had to think about that.

Her voice was gone. Marie was only able to whisper, which was very inconvenient and impractical. How should she go grocery shopping? She hated these impersonal supermarkets. For as long as she could think she had always been going to her bakery, her butcher's shop and the little store around the corner for the other things she needed. They didn't have self-service. She needed to tell the people what she wanted. She couldn't call her doctor either, which meant that she had to wait about four hours at the doctor's office. Marie sighed and touched her throat. Funny. It didn't actually hurt. Soon after, she was on her way to her doctor.

"It's laryngitis, Mrs. Dressler. That is very clear. How on earth did you do that? Dr. Schubert looked at her. "Well, we'll leave it for now and talk about it when you can talk again. He burst out laughing as though he had made a good joke. Then he prescribed drugs. Marie took the prescription, nodded, and left.

Her laryngitis was improving day by day. In the beginning she still was so hoarse that she hardly recognized her own voice, but now she could almost speak in normal volume again, although it still didn't sound healthy. If her health kept on improving like this, she would be able to call her rescuer soon. Luckily, he had given her his business card. She had a surprise for him.

The laryngitis had disappeared. Even without the drugs. Marie had put them aside after reading the package insert with all the side effects. There was no need to go through that. After all, she wasn't a spring chicken any more. She called the young man and arranged to meet with him.

"Pardon me? What did you say?" Hagen had real hearing problems. It wasn't particularly noisy in the small café, but he had difficulties understanding what the woman wanted to tell him. "I said that for several years I have only been at the house shortly just to check on things. I haven't been doing anything to the bungalow for quite some time and weeds run riot. But the landscape is beautiful. The house is located directly at the lake and it has its own dock. Marie hesitated for a moment. "I would be happy if you liked it. You are the right person for it." She looked at him expectantly. "What?" Hagen was at a loss of words. "You are really a little deaf, aren't you?" Now, Marie looked worried. "You should go and see a doctor soon. At your young age, you shouldn't take these things lightly." But Hagen smiled. This time, he had heard very well what she said.

"No, no, I heard everything. But I don't think I fully understood. Why do you want me to have the piece of land? And on top of that, you want to give it to me as a present?" Marie shrugged her shoulders. "That is very simple. I can't look after the property any longer and my sister can't either. We don't have any children. If we both dropped dead tomorrow the state would get everything. But I would like to give it to someone who can appreciate it. You are such a person, I am sure of that." She leaned back in her chair.

Hagen had a sip of his coffee. "But you don't know the first thing about me," he replied. He was still trying to process the things she had said. Actually, it had always been his dream to have a small piece of land at a lake with a dock where he could row out on the lake and fish for hours without anybody disturbing him. And now he should get it just like that. Marie smiled. "Of course I know you. I already made an appointment with the notary. Would tomorrow afternoon at 3:00 p.m. work for you?" Hagen nodded; he was still a little confused. "Of course, that works fine."

Conflict and Resolution

During the mugging, Marie suffered a fear-due-to-shock conflict. In the conflict active phase, ulcers, that is, a cell decrease, developed in the larynx, which she didn't notice. Sometimes there is minor pain, but the person rarely notices it consciously.

When Marie entered the healing phase – she had resolved the conflict – the mucosa swelled in order to balance the tissue loss, which resulted in hoarseness and partly even in the loss of her voice, respectively. She contracted a classic laryngitis.

The TB she and her family members had contracted after the war was, by the way, a healing after lung cancer, that is, a fear-of-death conflict.

The signs of palsy her mother experienced were the result of a motor conflict she suffered when she couldn't help her brother, Marie's uncle. She wanted to fend off the soldiers and hold them back, but she couldn't do it, because she didn't want to put her children at risk. So, her arms were partly paralyzed during the conflict active phase. A seizure must have occurred during the healing phase. Often it goes unnoticed, because it happens during sleep.

Hagen will continue to have problems with his hearing for a while, as he did suffer a hearing conflict at court because he couldn't believe what the judge was saying during his sentencing. The resolution of the conflict happened not too long ago, so that he will still experience hardness of hearing during the healing phase.

A Run For Life

• Jakob and leukemia

"I am faster than you," Jakob exclaimed and started running as fast as his feet would carry him. The boy could run like a greyhound. His father had a hard time keeping up with him. "I will get you," he gasped nonetheless and started running. He enjoyed doing the training with his son. Of course he could outrun him if he wanted to, but Jakob was really fast. He just turned 8 but he was a running talent. Gasping, the father was running side by side with the boy. "What would you say if we participated in the summer run? It is next week. We could run the two kilometers. What do you think?" Jakob looked at him, his eyes beaming. "And I will be the winner. Will I get a gold medal?" "Sure," promised his father. "If you win. But if not that wouldn't be a big deal either, right?" "I am sure that I will win," Jakob boasted and suddenly picked up the pace. He wanted to leave his father behind on the last meters.

"Jakob is very ambitious, hopefully he won't be too frustrated if someone else is faster than him," Jakob's mother pointed out that evening. Tina had been watching her two men very closely for quite some time now and she knew that Jakob always wanted to win at any cost. It worried her. "No worries," Daniel said and dismissed her concern. "Jakob can deal with it. And, what is more, he has to learn that he can't win all the time."

With the run approaching, Jakob trained even more obstinately. Every second day he ran with his father through the forest. Sometimes they took a longer route, sometimes a shorter one, but they rarely ran the same distance. If Daniel wanted to slow him down in order to prevent him from overtraining, Jakob protested. "Dad, I can keep running forever. I am not exhausted at all," he grouched. And when Daniel insisted, Jakob sometimes continued to run all by himself, which angered his parents.

Jakob was feverishly awaiting the run. He had marked the day in the calendar. Every day he scratched another day. The white spaces leading to his big day became fewer and fewer. "Sure I'll win," he assured his friend Nino. "I am the fastest." Nino didn't really listen. He wasn't interested in running. He didn't understand what could possibly be the fun of it. Soccer, yes, that was something else. But running?

Sunday, the day of the summer run, had arrived. Jakob was skipping nervously at the start line. Girls and boys were standing around him. Some of them were his age, but many were older. Most of them were about 10 years old. That didn't matter to Jakob. He would get them all. When the starter's gun fired, he started running as fast as he could. His father had told him to pace himself, but Jakob had forgotten all about it. Two kilometers were peanuts and he had to win after all.

He forged ahead immediately. He ignored the steps behind him and the breathing and gasping. He was running easily and he was feeling energetic. When he looked behind he saw that the distance between him and the others was growing. He was satisfied and concentrated on the route. He had finished half of the first round when he heard steps coming closer. He looked behind and saw a girl who had broken free from the other runners.

The girl was closely behind him. She was older than him with long legs and a steady pace. Jakob clenched his teeth. He exerted himself and picked up the pace further. That drained his energy. He could feel his heart beating in his ears and his legs turned to jelly. And he had run just one kilometer.

The girl stayed persistently behind him. She breathed evenly and didn't seem to be particularly exerted. The race took part only between the two of them. The main field was already 30 meters behind them. Jakob realized that he was in serious trouble. He couldn't keep up the pace for very much longer.

They had finished one and a half kilometers and just half a kilometer to run. At that point, the girl started the final spurt. With a steady pace she caught up to him, then she was running beside him, and in the next moment she had passed him. Only a few meters left to the line. The spectators cheered for the runners. Jakob's father shouted something, but Jakob didn't hear anything. He tried desperately to catch up with the girl again. Obstinately, he fought for every centimeter. It was in vain. The girl was the first to cross the finishing line; Jakob followed two meters behind her. He ran into his father's arms, crying.

Nothing could comfort Jakob. No matter what Daniel told him, Jakob didn't want to hear it. He didn't care that the girl was two years older than him and, therefore, had two more years of training. He also didn't care that he was second and had gotten the silver medal.

He had had a fight with Nino, who had teased him about the fact that a girl had beaten him. Jakob didn't want to run any more. Slowly, he walked through the city. He kept to himself and didn't talk very much. Tina reproached Daniel severely and said, "He desperately needs a success. I knew he would take it hard." Daniel was helpless. How could he restore a sense of achievement in Jakob?

Meanwhile, Jakob continued to suffer. One day, when he was once again gloomily moping through the streets, a boy came running out of a cigarette store. He was maybe 13 or 14 years old. An old man came limping after him. "Stop, you have to pay first. Don't run away, boy." The boy didn't care about the old man at all. He turned around and showed him the finger. In his other hand he held a carton of Marlboro.

Almost without Jakob realizing it, his feet started moving. He was running faster and faster. Like a little greyhound he ran after the boy, who was at least two heads taller than Jakob. But he was a lame duck, Jakob decided.

He enjoyed the race. He came closer and closer to the thief. The passers-by got out of his way; behind him, the old man kept shouting something Jakob didn't understand. He had almost caught up with the thief. Apparently, he had heard Jakob approaching. He turned around and when he saw Jakob, he looked surprised. "Hey kiddo, what do you want from me?" Then he picked up the pace a little. But he was too slow for Jakob. Without a word, he jumped at the thief from behind and held his legs, so that he fell down. Lying on top of him, Jakob looked around for help.

The thief was so perplexed that he reacted too late. When he wanted to shake Jakob off, eventually, a man had already grabbed him by the shoulders, turned his arms on his back and took the cigarettes from him. A second man used his cell phone to call the police. Jakob got up, cleaned the dust from his pants, and looked around. At least six grown-ups were standing around him and gazed at him. Finally, the man who had called the police gave him a pat on the back. "You are a super fast runner. I haven't seen someone running as fast as you in a while."

Jakob was proud when he showed his father the Swiss pocket knife the store owner had given him as a thank you. Tina stifled her doubts about the gift for an eight year old. The beaming expression on her son's face was more important to her. "So, buddy," his father said, "are we going to continue our training tomorrow?" Jakob grinned. "Sure, but you don't have a chance beating me anyway."

The knee hurt terribly. First, Jakob didn't want to tell his father about it. But how should he explain that he simply couldn't do the training. They had just started running again two weeks ago. And he had become better and better. They regularly ran a distance of five kilometers. Jakob had to tell his father. The pain couldn't continue like this.

Daniel stopped the training for the time being. When Jakob's condition didn't improve after a week, Tina put her foot down. She took her son to the doctor. The knee was x-rayed and the doctor had a strange look on his face when he sent them back to their family doctor. "It looks like Jakob has leukemia," he said unmoved while he was writing a referral. "Take this and go to the hospital. They will take care of it."

Tina was shocked. Leukemia? Where did that suddenly come from? Jakob had heard the word before. A boy who lived in the house across the street had leukemia. He was in the hospital for weeks already. The last time Jakob had seen him he was bald. And in school they had said that he was probably going to die. "Mom, what is leukemia," Jakob asked. Tina looked at him, ran her hand over his hair, and said, "We will find out."

Conflict and Resolution

Jakob suffered a collapse of his self-esteem connected to his athletic performance when the girl outran him and prevented him from winning the race. The Hamer Focus (HH) for this Dirk Hamer syndrome (DHS) is located in the white matter of the cerebrum. In the conflict active phase there is the occurrence of osteolyses, that is, a sell decrease in the affected part of the skeleton.

When Jakob was praised for being so fast during the chasing of the thief and even received a gift, his conflict was resolved. In the healing phase occurs a bone edema, which stretches the periosteum. The holes in the bone are being filled again or also recalcified.

The number of blood cells increases again, after they decreased in the conflict active phase. The traditional medicine talks about leukemia. Leukemia is the healing phase after a collapse of self-esteem. It is very painful in the affected areas. But, above all, it causes a lot of fear.

In the sense of the traditional, traditional medicine, leukemia is considered a life-threatening disease. Consequently, many patients are systematically treated to death with chemotherapy and radiation.

The important thing for people who suffered such a collapse of their self-esteem is that they are patient. Talking about the experience and taking light pain relievers makes the healing easier. The meaning of the pain during the healing phase is to immobilize the affected part of the body, because it is especially susceptible to breaking during this time.

A Chance For Paul
• Irene and the lungs

Irene was shocked when she looked into the sink. She saw the blood that she had just coughed up. Her blood ran cold. She had worried about it. The whole time she felt that something was wrong. And now her feeling was confirmed. She was coughing up blood. Her legs were weak. Sapless, she shuffled into the living room. She fell into the couch and just stared. It was just too much at once.

"Mrs. Handtke, please," the voice in the speaker of the waiting room resounded. She got up and walked into the doctor's room. She didn't expect anything but clarification. She knew the doctor for a dozen years, but he was still as strange as he had been the first day. He hastily said hello, then he picked up a sheet of paper, pretended to immerse himself in the letter, and then lifted his head and looked at her. She looked back at him calmly.

"I am sorry to tell you that we have found lung nodules. That means you have lung cancer. We suspect that they are metastases from your ovary cancer." He paused as though he was waiting for a reaction. When Irene nodded, he continued a little insecure, "We can't do much more. We recommend chemotherapy and radiation, but we can't tell whether it will help." He put the piece of paper aside and looked at her again. Irene nodded again. Then she got up. "Thank you, but I don't think I want to go through that again. It is not right." She cut off his protest with a gesture of her hand. Then she turned around and left.

She made St. John's wort tea. It reminded her of her childhood. Often, she had spent her holidays at her grandmother's. In the summer they had picked St. John's wort, huge bunches. Part of it they had made into tea right away and the rest they had hung to dry in the attic. She closed her eyes and smelled the aroma. Then she had a sip of the hot, red brew and enjoyed the taste. Something rubbed up against her legs. Automatically, she ran her hand over her cat's back. Fridolin always knew when she needed some comfort. At the time her husband had suddenly collapsed and no one could help him any more, Fridolin had kept an eye on her for weeks.

Fred had died so quickly, that she still couldn't believe it. It happened so unexpected and they had had a fight only few hours before. They had made up only halfway when it happened.

It had taken her months to get over it. She couldn't let go of the self-reproaches until her son became a father. A smile went over her face. Little Paul instantly reminded her of Fred. "As if he was born again," she had remarked when she saw the little face. Her son had looked at her in surprise, "You are right, he actually looks like him."

André had been very close with his father. He had been a real father's boy. Even as an adult he would go to his father when there was a problem. He was devastated by his father's death. So much so, that Irene had to deal not only with her own pain but also with the constant worry about André. And if that wasn't enough, one morning she had detected a lump in her right breast.

At first, she panicked, but then she simply suppressed the thought of the lump. "I had too many other things on my mind," she remembered now, while she had another sip of her tea. "And that was exactly right," she concluded in hindsight. Initially, it seemed as though the lump had grown, but when she didn't think about it any more and didn't go to the doctor either, it wasn't important for her any more.

Now it was gone. She couldn't remember how that had happened. She couldn't feel it any longer. Absent-mindedly, she examined her breast. Nothing was there any more.

But something else had appeared. At first she had experienced lower abdominal pain. It had alarmed her and her responsibility as a new grandmother had caused her to see a doctor. The diagnosis had shocked her. "Ovarian cancer," the doctor, who she didn't know, had told her laconically. It was a malignant cyst. Then they gave her an appointment for surgery. She clearly remembered the moment when she woke up again. "We sent the tissue to the lab to have it examined. We decide how to proceed when we get the results back." And three days later, the doctor broke the news to her that the cyst had been malignant. "Your only option is chemotherapy and radiation. Prophylactic, in order to prevent metastases."

Irene's tea had got cold. She put the cup aside and, lost in thought, ruffled the cat's fur. She drifted into pondering again. What was she supposed to do now? She had already put this treatment behind her once and she had sworn she wouldn't do that to herself again. For weeks, she had been suffering from nausea and pain, she had lost her hair, and her weight went down to 48 kilos. Her normal weight was 65 kilos. The way her neighbours had looked at her constantly worried her and her son had this expression of panic on his face. He had supported and encouraged her. "But we need you, mom," he had said. "Paul wants to get to know his grandmother." So she had come through.

And it did look promising. As if she had overcome the disease. And now she had this cough and the doctor said it was lung cancer. She shook her head, got up, and took the photo album out of the armoire. Then she immersed herself into the pictures of Fred and herself, of André when he was a child, pictures of her parents and grandparents. What was she supposed to do?

"No, I won't do that," she vigorously repeated the sentence her family doctor didn't want to hear. "But, Mrs. Handtke, you won't survive if you refuse the treatment," he objected. "You have to have this therapy, otherwise no one can help you." But Irene remained firm. "I have sworn to myself that I won't endure that ordeal again. You won't change my mind." Then she hung up.

Relieved, she had a look around. Then she took the bags, which were already packed, grabbed the carrier with Fridolin and got into the car. She would spend the last weeks and month at her newly bought vacation home in Spain. André would visit her regularly together with his family. That was definite.

"Granny, how did you feel when grandpa died?" asked Paul and looked at her. Her grandson was coming along well. The little boy had turned into a serious and thoughtful ten year old. He was curious and inquisitive. Irene looked at him. "As if I had lost the most precious thing in my life, and as if I hadn't shown him often enough how I felt about him. It was terrible. But then you were born and that gave me some comfort. You instantly reminded me of him." She gave him a big hug. In the backyard, Paul's sister, Nele, screamed with laughter. She had brought two friends. Irene didn't mind that at all, the more activity the better.

"And when you got sick with that serious disease? Did you think about dying?" Paul looked at her inquiringly. Fridolin sat on his lap; he was getting old and, since, preferred his peace. Thus, he got along better with Paul than with Nele. "Naturally, I did," Irene replied. "First I was very scared of dying. After all, I had you, my grandson, who needed his granny. Throughout the treatment I couldn't stop panicking."

She was silent for a moment. Then she said, "You know, when I had overcome the serious disease they suddenly diagnosed another one that was even more serious." Paul had a shocked expression on his face. "You never told me." "I haven't told your father either, said Irene.

Now, Paul looked even more surprised. "You don't have to tell everything. Sometimes, talking about it makes things even worse," Irene explained. "It was good for me that I simply didn't do anything. I took a long vacation here in Spain together with Fridolin. For several weeks I had a bad cough and was all in a sweat during the nights. Sometimes I had to change the sheets three times."

Lost in thoughts, she looked out of the window. "I know, grandma, it was the same with me when I had pyelitis. Mom always had to get new sheets." Paul nodded gravely and petted Fridolin. Irene turned around, cleared the plates from the table, which they had used to have some fruit, and answered, "Yes, and after a few month I felt much better. I felt up to anything."

She laughed. "The doctors who later examined me again didn't find anything. They talked about a miracle." Irene grinned to herself. "Well, was it a miracle?" Paul asked. Irene shrugged her shoulders. "I doubt that these doctors know what a miracle is." Then she looked at her watch, squinted against the sun, and picked up a book. "We have pondered enough. I will have my siesta now."

Conflict and Resolution

Irene suffered three DHSs. The first one occurred when her husband Fred died suddenly and unexpectedly. She suffered a severe conflict of loss, which caused tissue loss in one ovary during the conflict active phase.

At the same time, she was very worried about her son and how he would cope with his father's death. In the conflict active phase, this worry conflict triggered breast cancer in her right breast, as she is left-handed. If she had been right-handed, the lump would have appeared in her left breast, which, then, would have been her mother/child side, and the right side of her body would have been the partner side. She largely ignored the breast cancer and when her grandson was born, who reminded her of her husband, the severe conflict of loss she suffered first was resolved.

The process of developing necrosis stopped in the respective areas and the holes were filled again. An ovarian cyst occurred, which first grows attached to the surrounding organs and later detaches again if the person awaits further developments. In Irene's case, the ovaries were removed beforehand.

But the cancer diagnoses triggered a fear-of-death conflict, which presented itself in the form of lung nodules. After the treatment and the apparent healing, the conflict was resolved and the nodules healed through caseating. The coughing of blood is a sign that the lung cancer is healing. This is the phase where most people go to see the doctor. That's how Irene's lung cancer was diagnosed as well.

Her breast cancer healed with the birth of her grandson also because she didn't have to worry about her son any longer. In this case, the lump decomposed without her really noticing it. The ovarian cancer was only detected, because it grows in the conflict resolved- or healing phase and, thus, is considered malignant according to the traditional opinion. She didn't have the lung cancer treated, so it could heal undisturbed while she was in Spain.

Skin-to-Skin Contact
• Ruth and the neurodermatitis

Furiously, he stomped into the bathroom where his wife was dressing Julia's eczemas with bandages and hissed, "When do I actually get to see you except late at night when you fall fast asleep in a matter of seconds." Ruth clenched her teeth, "Not now, Bernd, let's talk about this later. I still have to treat David and then I'll put them to bed." Bernd flashed his eyes at her. "Well, just send them to bed and get them out of the way." He stomped out of the bathroom.

Ruth listened as the fridge door was opened; then it sizzled. Bernd got himself a beer. Ruth sighed. What was she supposed to do? On the one hand, she had to take care of the business and Bernd wasn't any help in that department. He constantly made mistakes, which she had to smooth away again later on. At home with the children he wasn't very helpful either. Obviously, he didn't feel well. "When I am grown up I will help you, mom." Julia looked up at her with big eyes and smiled. "I am sure I won't have the bad rash any more either. And neither does David. And then, dad can do everything he wants to do."

Ruth gave her daughter a kiss on the nose while she attached the end of the last bandage. The little girl had another bad neurodermatitis episode. And so did David. The children would scratch the affected spots until they were bleeding if she didn't dress them. By dressing them, she could at least prevent that from happening if she couldn't prevent the symptoms. The disease started five years ago, at the same time she started the business and was busy all the time, when she came to think of it. Nobody had been able to help so far. She had consulted every doctor and specialist and had tried every therapy and several different diets, but the success was only short-lived.

During the cure, both children had hardly any problems. They had been away for six weeks. And although Ruth had a hard time leaving the business, she enjoyed the reduced stress. No double shift working in the business and at home for a change. She felt a lot better. Unfortunately, the symptoms had become worse than before after they returned. The episode was so bad, that they had hot, red, and itchy patches all over their entire body. "As though would have an allergic reaction against me," Ruth thought. She put Julia to bed. "I'll read you a story in just a moment." Then she took David to the bathroom.

"It can't go on like this, Ruth." Bernd was walking back and forth through the room. Meanwhile he had changed to Whiskey. "You have no time for the family any more. The business is the most important thing for you. We don't get to see you at all. And every now and then I want to do something else then be the babysitter." Ruth looked at him; she ran her hand across her forehead. "And who will put the food on the table if I give up the business? Am I supposed to stay home and you look for a job?" A sneer appeared on her face but disappeared again immediately. Bernd had noticed it. He stopped, "That's exactly what we will do. We will give up the business, I will find a job, and you stay at home with the children. Maybe then they will get better for a change." He put down his glass angrily, turned around and left the room. She listened as he closed the front door behind him.

It would have been nice to just forget about all the problems. But she knew that that wouldn't work. Not with Bernd. He didn't have any perseverance, quit every job after a short time, and was simply incapable of providing for the family. Therefore, Ruth had to keep the ball rolling business-wise. And, in addition, she had to keep struggling with her husband.

"If the kids could at least get rid of the neurodermatitis," she thought. It was really strange. When she was at seminars, on business trips, or at a lecture, they obviously felt better. Full of enthusiasm, they would tell her on the phone that their itchy patches were almost gone, but as soon as she returned home and wanted to see the miracle, it was over. Every time, Julia and David suffered another neurodermatitis episode. It didn't improve at all.

The next day she decided that they needed a brief vacation. She arranged everything with her secretary, gave her the most important appointments, and said goodbye, "See you next week." Julia and David were thrilled. Instead of a boring sick day they would spend the day together with her mother. Even a whole week! Both were excited and ran around the room shouting, "We are going to the zoo!" "We have to see the new baby elephant," Julia said. Bernd didn't look so happy. "I won't come with you. If you are home, I can finally go and see my buddies for a change. Haven't seen them in ages."

Tired and exhausted, Julia and David fell into their beds. Ruth had applied the ointment to their affected patches of skin and had dressed them in order to prevent the children from scratching. Luckily, they didn't notice the pitiful looks of the other visitors who had stared at their eczemas on their arms and faces. No, it hadn't improved. It had become even worse. It hurt Ruth to see her children suffer. But she just didn't know how to help them.

"Are you sure?" Bernd looked surprised after all. "As sure as I can be. I will get a partner and retire from the business. And you will get a job, but not in my company. I don't want you to interfere with the man." Ruth's voice sounded resolute. Bernd swallowed. Actually, he had hoped to play the boss. That was typical for Ruth to spoil the party. But he knew that he wouldn't be able to change her mind. "OK, so I will start looking for a job." After all, that was better than being the nurse for the kids. At least, he would meet other people.

"You will stay home, mom? And what happens with your business?" Julia was torn between worry and enthusiasm. Ruth reassured her. "I found someone who knows a lot about the business. He will be the director," she explained. "And we can be together every day?" David looked at her as if she was Santa Clause. The six year old would start school this year. Julia was already in grade 2. "Yes, we can. And when you have to go to school I will wait here at home until you come back." David's face was beaming. Then he ran through the apartment, turned somersaults, and let off howls of joy. Ruth laughed. It was nice to be so welcome.

At first, her exclusive role as a mother wasn't easy for her. She repeatedly caught herself wanting to call at the company to give instructions. Several times, she had already picked up the receiver, but then stopped herself.

The course of her children's neurodermatitis was also discouraging for her. It just wouldn't get better. First, they seemed to suffer even more severe episodes than before. Sometimes, Ruth wanted to cry out of helplessness.

Only Bernd surprised her in a positive way. He had found a job as an engineer in a building company. And this time, he seemed to be successful.

After the first three weeks, Ruth saw for the first time some light at the end of the tunnel. The skin of Julia and David seemed to improve. The red, itchy patches disappeared more and more. She didn't need either ointment or other drugs. Two days ago they had still been there, yesterday they saw fewer of them, and today they were almost gone. The two of them really flourished. And when David started school there was nothing that distinguished him from his future classmates. He had clear, rosy skin; the eczema was history.

Crying, David came running towards her. Ruth's heart almost stopped. "Where have you been? Julia isn't home either; I am all by myself. Have you gone back to work again? Why did you leave me alone?" David cried. He fell into her arms and suddenly started yelling, "Why didn't you say anything." Ruth calmed him down, talked to him in a quiet voice, and ran her hand over his hair. "I just had to get some eggs. I didn't know you were coming home so early. Did they let you go an hour early today?"

Gradually, David calmed down. He was able to tell her that her teacher had suddenly gotten sick and they were allowed to go home earlier. Ruth frowned. That was unusual; the school had to notify the parents of the first graders about cancelled classes and had to supervise the children in the meantime. She had to clarify that with the principal. But first of all she would prepare lunch.

Only a few hours later and David couldn't stop scratching. He scratched his arms and his neck like mad. The eczema appeared everywhere. He had a severe relapse. Julia was all right. She didn't have any problems. Ruth treated David with the ointment and dressed the affected areas. Then she sighed in frustration. It would probably never stop. Obviously, David thought the same thing. "I want it to stop. Why do I have eczema and the other kids in my class don't?" Ruth shrugged her shoulders. "If I just knew...."

Conflict and Resolution

Both children suffered a separation conflict when they saw their mother, to whom they are obviously very attached, less and less. They experienced the DHS very early at the time when she opened her business and had to take care of it. Assumingly, the father wasn't perceived and accepted as her replacement.

During the conflict active phase the skin develops barely visible necroses. The skin is less sensitive to pain, but also overall less sensitive. During the conflict resolved phase these necroses are being filled; swelling and redness appear and the skin is itching. Whenever the children had contact with her mother again, they entered the healing phase and, thus, apparently had another episode. When the mother was gone, even for days, the eczema disappeared almost completely. The children seemed to be healed, but they were actually in the conflict active phase. The mother's decision to stay at home triggered the final healing for them. But David suffered a relapse when he came home and his mother wasn't there. His body reacted respectively as he hit a track.

Neurodermatitis can affect all areas of the skin; however, often only those are affected that had the most contact with the beloved person or animal, that is, the face, the hands, the head, and the back. Neurodermatitis can also be the result of a separation conflict involving a pet. In that case, many people develop neurodermatitis in areas where they petted the animal. If a person petted a cat primarily at its head and back, he or she will more that likely develop neurodermatitis at his or her head or back.

In many cases doctors diagnose a cat allergy, because it is conspicuous that these people develop their eczema while being in contact with cats. As a matter of fact, the body that hits a track reacts with an alarm and a quick all-clear as soon as it realizes that the situation is harmless. The conflict resolution then presents itself in the form of neurodermatitis.

Spa Romance
• Frank and the kidneys

"Well, you will have to exercise a little bit, you have added quite a few pounds, buddy." With a knowing look, Rainer tapped on Frank's belly, which had become rather conspicuous. Frank had a weary smile on his face when he walked over to his locker. "Exercise? And what else am I supposed to do?" he asked himself angrily. Three times a week he jogged about five kilometers and twice a week he went bowling. Admittingly, that wasn't too exhausting, but it didn't explain the fact that, instead of losing weight, he had gained 15 kilos within the last six months. He couldn't look at himself in the mirror any more. "Actually, it doesn't really matter," he thought with a grim sense of humour. "Kerstin left me, so it doesn't matter how I look."

Kerstin had left him helter-skelter after a big fight four months ago. She moved out over night and had left him behind all alone. It came unexpected for Frank. They had fought a lot, but it had been unimaginable for him that she would leave him just like that.

The reason had actually been of no significance. She had asked him to accompany her to a lecture she was giving at her niece's school. It was about some kind of psycho stuff for teachers. She was very nervous and he promised her to come. But he completely forgot about it. He went for a beer with his friends and simply didn't think about it any more. Kerstin had left the same evening.
Around the same time, he was laid off. The company was cutting jobs again for internal reasons. This time it was his turn. He shouldn't have been surprised, but he was anyway. "It is quite a different thing to experience it personally," Frank thought and tied his sneakers.

He had problems bending down because his belly was in the way. But he had also gained weight at his legs, arms; his entire body had become heavier.

Frank remembered that he had been overweight when he was a child. It had been terrible for him. Everybody had teased him. He had always been the target for mockery and nasty pranks. His older brother had to defend him all the time. No day went by without Eckehard getting into a fight because of him. Until his parents sent him for treatment to a sanatorium. The timing was good. He lost weight and thanks to a growth period that followed he didn't put the weight back on again. He had enjoyed being slim. Frank sighed when he thought back. "Maybe I should go to a sanatorium again."

It had been four weeks since Frank had started his treatment at the sanatorium. After his doctor had constantly pestered him about it and, furthermore, had diagnosed him with gout in the early stage, Frank had agreed to take treatment in a sanatorium. And to his surprise it worked out.

He had mixed feelings when he went to the small village in the mountains and admitted himself to the clinic. But in the meantime he really liked it there. He had a strict schedule. Every morning he had to exercise moderately. Then he went for breakfast and afterwards everybody had his or her special therapies. In the afternoon, they attended group sessions. Frank wasn't quite sure what they were good for as all of the patients were here because of physical problems. But then again, the talking made him feel good too.

"Would you like to accompany me to the post office? I need some stamps." Dagmar's question had sounded innocent, yet Frank was a little excited. "Like a teenager," he thought and laughed about himself. He was surprised, though, that Dagmar had asked him. She would have been "Miss Clinic" if that title had existed. She was in her mid-thirties, slim with blond hair, athletic, and pretty. All the men looked at her wishfully whereas the women looked envious. Frank never thought that she would want to get to know him. "Sure, I'd love to," he answered quickly. They arranged to meet in the afternoon.

"You have gout? You are too young for that." Dagmar was surprised. Frank shrugged his shoulders. "I am almost 40, which isn't that young any more. At any rate, I don't know what could be the reason. Nobody knows for sure if you know what I mean. The doctors just make assumptions."

Dagmar nodded thoughtfully. "That's right. I have had my back pain for years without any improvement. That's why I ended up here." "And is it getting better?" Frank looked at her curiously. Dagmar shrugged her shoulders. "I don't know. At first it seemed to improve, although the pain is coming back again now. We'll see. But it is definitely nice to go for a walk with you. That's at least something, right?" She looked at him mischievously.

Frank blushed. Quickly, he looked to the side. "I already feel much better," he changed the subject. That was right, when he came to think of it. He didn't have any gout pain, but then again, he only had had pain in his big toe once before, and the doctor just assumed possible problems. However, he had a Woolworth's bladder lately. He had to use the washroom all the time. It was almost embarrassing. He laughed. "Are you laughing about me or at me?" asked Dagmar, a little insecure. "Always laughing at you," Frank replied. Then he kissed her softly on the cheek. He felt like a teenager.

He urgently needed a painkiller. His toe hurt terribly. "Gout attack," was the doctor's diagnose. "You have to avoid meat and such for now. I am going to prepare a respective diet for you." Frank clenched his teeth and took the painkiller. The pain brought tears to his eyes.

He didn't tell Dagmar about the attack. He was embarrassed. Frank didn't want to be old. Least of all, when he was with Dagmar. Their relationship was promising.

"You will move in with me and then you start looking for a job," Dagmar said convincingly. "Are you sure you want that?" Frank hesitated. "Yes, I am sure. Maybe you should keep your apartment for a while, just in case you find out that you were wrong about your feelings for me." He looked shocked. "Don't look at me like that," she laughed and gave him a little punch in the side." "It is good to be prepared."

Frank was thankful. The first time in his life it occurred to him how lucky he was. Three months had passed since they had returned from the sanatorium. Two months ago, he and Dagmar had moved in together and it worked out great.

He had found a lucrative job he enjoyed and had lost weight without really noticing it. He had suffered one more gout attack shortly before he moved in with Dagmar, but after that the problems disappeared.

Dagmar's back pain had improved as well. First, she had had several incidents where the pain was bad, but in the meantime the pain had disappeared.

He realized that he had lost weight, about five kilos in six weeks although he didn't work out more than before. As a matter of fact, he worked out less. And he ate a lot more. It struck him as strange that, before, he had eaten a few pieces of vegetable once a day. Together with Dagmar, he had three meals a day and was still losing weight. He didn't understand it, but it was certainly OK with him.

Deep inside, Frank stayed on alert. He didn't want to fall in a black hole again as was the case when Kerstin left him. At first, he started every day thinking that things could change again quickly. It was only after some time had gone by that he was able to relax. "And even if things should change," he thought. "That's life. I will enjoy the moment. If it doesn't work out, I can deal with it. But life always goes on somehow."

Conflict and Resolution

Frank suffered a refugee conflict when he lost his job. Although he should have expected it, he didn't see it coming and was completely overwhelmed.

The refugee- or existence conflict includes the aspect of "having lost everything," "feeling like being bombed out," or "being thrown out of one's apartment or home country." It results in the development of a compact tumor of the kidney tubular cells during the conflict active phase, which obstructs or blocks the urine flow of the respective kidney. If, at the same time, the person is in the healing phase regarding another conflict, the healing edema of that particular conflict increases.

The body accumulates an extreme amount of excess fluid; before long, the person gains a lot of weight. Frank suffered an additional collapse of self-esteem involving his foot, but it is in the healing phase, which manifests itself in a so-called gout attack. Gout is a combination of an active kidney tubular conflict and a resolved collapse of self-esteem, often involving the big toe or the knee, but seldom other joints.

The collapse of self-esteem was connected to Kerstin. He had promised to accompany her to the lecture, but he didn't go. His feeling was that he "should have gone." Biologically spoken, he had failed with his foot. He suffered a foot-activity collapse of self-esteem with gout occurring in his big toe. He suddenly realized psychologically that he made a mistake, and how much she meant to him. Frank resolved the conflict when he found a new job. He lost the accumulated fluid that had bloated him by virtually peeing it out.

Dagmar had a collapse of self-esteem in the healing phase, which manifested itself in back pain. As the pain repeatedly recurred, she probably hit a track. The problem was possibly connected to men, because her back pain occurred very often during her treatment at the sanatorium where all the men were admiring her. It is quite possible that she was rejected at one point and, thus, suffered a collapse of self-esteem.

The Cat Blues
• Julian and non-Hodgkin's lymphoma

Julian was heartbroken. For hours he had been crying in his room. Every now and then he stopped only to start again after a few minutes. Julian was 12 years old. At that age boys don't want to get caught crying. That's why he hadn't left his room all day. He had skipped school today; he just didn't care. His parents didn't know about it yet, but they would soon find out. But Julian didn't care about that either. He didn't want to see or hear from anybody. Julian cried for his little tomcat. Feivel was dead. Julian still couldn't believe it. For one week they had been fighting for his life. The courageous little cat, which was just one year old and not fully-grown yet, didn't give up that easily. But in the end, he didn't make it.

Julian started sobbing louder again. A week ago, Feivel had been hit by a car. The speed limit was only 30km per hour, but hardly anybody paid attention to that. And Feivel was young and inexperienced. Instead of roaming in the surrounding gardens, he was always drawn to the other side of the street to the old industrial site.

Julian had trusted his little tomcat. He was smart, nothing would happen to him. But then it did happen. A neighbour was at the door, " There is a cat lying on the street. It is hurt. I think it's yours." Julian couldn't forget those words. He had been sick to his stomach. The blood had left his cheeks and he ran to the spot the neighbour had mentioned.

Feivel was lying on his side. Blood came out of his mouth, but he was still alive. Julian picked him up carefully. Tears were in his eyes. Very gently he carried Feivel over to their apartment. Then he called his mother. She had to take Feivel to the vet immediately.

"It doesn't look good. His lungs are hurt and he probably has other internal injuries as well. I wouldn't let him suffer any longer." Julian was furious at the vet. "You don't even know how severe his injuries are and you want to kill him? What kind of a doctor are you?" His eyes were full of tears again, but this time they were partly tears of anger. His mother put her arm around his shoulder to calm him down. "Dr. Kremer just wants to help Feivel. Please calm down."

Feivel was lying on the examination table. Apparently, the pain reliever had helped him a little bit. He even purred for a moment when Julian petted him gently on its little head. Julian knew that cats would purr also from pain. His heart was heavy with worry. "We will take him home, right, mom? Maybe he will recover and he will get better soon. He will get well. I am sure he will. He just has to."

The fight for his live had lasted a week. Julian hadn't left Feivel's side. He kept petting him and couldn't help but imagine how Feivel must have felt when he saw the approaching car, mercilessly rolling towards him; it was much too fast and didn't stop. Feivel must have been paralyzed, unable to run away. And then it had hit him. At this point, Julian would always cover his face in his hands and start sobbing. He could physically feel the little cat's fear.

Feivel kept fighting for his life. After three days it seemed as though he would recover. He had even dragged himself to the water bowl. However, he didn't want to have any food. Julian started to feel optimistic only to have his hopes shattered a short time later. Already the next day Feivel suffered a relapse. He was just lying there, had trouble breathing, and didn't even lift his head when Julian was talking to him. After two more days he died. He had looked at Julian one more time and then he had passed away.

Feivel had a proper funeral. He was buried in the back yard under the apple tree. Julian had made him a coffin and didn't allow any comments. He didn't look at anybody while he was filling the grave of his cat with soil. His face looked grim.

That was all Julian needed. Not only was he at a loss about how he should go on without Feivel, but he also seemed to get sick. Again and again he had this dragging pain in his throat, a pinching under the skin. The doctor couldn't find anything. Julian just ignored the pain.

He really didn't want to come to this place. His parents had dragged him to the animal shelter. "Why would I go there?" Julian had grumbled. "No other cat can replace Feivel. No one can make him come back to me. And I really don't need an experience like that again." Eventually, they managed to get him into the car after all. "Not a replacement, we know that," his father had said. "But just consider this. All these cats are looking for a home. And maybe one of them will like you so much that it wants to stay with you. And if not, no harm done."

Now, Julian was standing there and his parents stole a glance at each other. He had a smile on his face they hadn't seen in quite a long time. The little red cat had come running towards Julian and curled its tail into a question mark. It had rubbed its little head against his legs and had started purring almost immediately.

"This cat was brought to us a few weeks ago. It's a girl. We call her 'Foxy'," explained the manager of the animal shelter. "Since she came here she and our Rambo have been inseparable." She pointed to a middle-sized black and white tomcat with tousled ears. "They can only go together. Otherwise they have to stay here."

Rambo looked over Julian suspiciously. Julian called him while he continued to pet Foxy. Rambo seemed to think for a moment before he came walking towards them. Foxy turned away from Julian shortly, said hello to Rambo, and licked his forehead. She groomed him for a little while and he obviously enjoyed it. Then she turned around again and strutted over to Julian. Rambo followed her.

"I just don't want to let them go outside. It is too dangerous." Julian furiously stamped his foot. His mother looked at him thoughtfully. "Life is dangerous, Julian. You can't prevent things from happening. But look at them. They need fresh air as much as you do. They need the grass and the rain, butterflies and bugs, they want to lie in the sun and tussle with other cats." Julian held his ears. "No, I don't want them to go outside." Rambo and Foxy looked at him motionless. Then they looked out of the window again.

Every noise of an engine had Julian wince. He could tell only by listening how fast a car was going. As always, most of them were too fast. Then he would run to the balcony and threatened them with his fist to go slower.

The last time his friend, René, had visited him he said, "Julian, you have bats in the belfry! Why are you getting so wound up? They won't drive slower just because of you." He thought Julian was a little crazy. "Maybe he is right," Julian thought. But since Foxy and Rambo were allowed to go outside – he couldn't resist their sad looks any longer – he worried all the time. His thoughts circled around cars and injured cats. He constantly saw monstrous wheels come rolling at him; he felt like a little cat that was unable to avoid the cars.

As soon as they closed the doors in the evenings after the cats had returned, Julian felt better. He was able to relax to a certain extent. But he knew it couldn't go on like this. Julian didn't believe in god, but now he started to pray. Someone, anyone, should do something to protect Rambo and Foxy.

Someone had heard Julian's prayers. He wouldn't have to worry about his cats any longer. At least not that much. They had installed speed bumps, so that car drivers couldn't go faster than 30km even if they wanted. They just crawled along the street, cursing. Such a speed bump could get nasty if a car was too fast. Julian grinned when he watched how carefully the drivers were going. It took a load off his mind. At this speed, not even a drunk could overlook a cat. And the cats wouldn't be too shocked to run away in time.

Foxy and Rambo lay in Julian's bed, purring. Startled, the boy touched his neck, which was hurting at the right side. In front of the ear directly under the skin he felt a big round lump. It hurt when Julian touched it. And further below, he could feel another one developing. He jumped up, ran into the bathroom, and looked at his neck in the mirror. It looked strange. Below the two round ones he saw a few more lumps like pearls on a necklace. But he could feel those ones rather than see them.

At dinner, his parents noticed them as well. "You hold your head on a angle, is something wrong?" his mother asked. She sounded worried. He showed her the lumps. "I detected them today. They hurt and I don't have any idea how they got there." His mother examined his neck carefully. It was Friday evening. "We'll see how it looks on Monday; maybe we have to see the doctor," she decided. Julian nodded carefully. A little later, he crawled into bed. He was too tired to watch TV today, and he didn't have the energy to read either. He fell asleep almost immediately. Foxy and Rambo snuggled closely against him.

"The lumps went down." His mother examined Julian's neck and was satisfied. "I think you can go back to school. If the neck hurts, just tell your teacher and come back home." Julian nodded. Then he yawned. "How are you feeling?" His mother was worried again immediately. "Just tired," Julian answered. Then he petted Foxy and Rambo's heads. Both of them rubbed against his legs.

"See you later," Julian said and walked out of the door. When he saw the big BMW crawling along the street with its driver carefully trying to avoid the speed bumps, Julian grinned. Still grinning, he made the victory sign.

Conflict and Resolution

Julian suffered a frontal fear conflict when his tomcat, Feivel, was hit by a car and was fighting for his life. Julian put himself in the shoes of the animal and experienced its fear in its place.

Even after the cat's death, Julian's thoughts kept circling around the fear; Julian was highly conflict active. During this phase, ulcers or tissue loss developed in the old brachial arch tubes that aren't in use any more. The boy noticed it only through mild dragging pain every once in a while.

The conflict remained active even with the two new cats he constantly worried about. He got onto a track. Only after the street was safer for the cats did the conflict resolve and Julian entered the healing phase.

The swelling during the healing phase caused fluid cysts, which are partly visible through the skin. These brachial arch fluid cysts are caused by severe swelling during the healing in the ulcerated areas of the disused tubes of the old brachial arches, which are lined with squamous epithelium mucosa.

Therefore, the fluid can't drain off and develops parts of raised tube pieces filled with fluid on both sides of the neck in front of and behind the ear, stretching further down towards the pit of the collarbone and they can reach up to the midriff. However, in most cases only one area is affected, that is, the cysts don't develop along the entire brachial arch tube. The traditional medicine would diagnose non-Hodgkin's at this point, a kind of lymph node cancer.

Below The Belt

• Karl and the prostrate

Motionlessly, Karl stared at the photos on the table in front of him, which he had found in the mail today. The letter had his address on it. Its content didn't leave any doubt. Ilona was cheating on him; apparently she had done so for quite some time. Her lover was a young guy. An athletic type who, in regards to his age, could easily be his son. Not much older than 28. Karl put his head in his hands. Then he had another look at the photos. It was his fault entirely. All his friends had warned him. "Don't get married to a woman who is so much younger than you. She will twist you around her little finger and hurt your feelings."

But what was he supposed to do. He had been hopelessly in love. So he married Ilona. She was 30 years his junior. And it had seemed as though she would love him too. How should he know better? He had been a bachelor for most of his life. Not unattractive, as many women had told him again and again. But he wouldn't commit to a long-term relationship. Not until he met Ilona.

He heard steps in the hallway. Karl lifted his head. "Hey honey," Ilona lilted and kissed him. He looked at her; he didn't try to hide the photos. She glanced at them. "Oh," she said. Then she picked one up. "You spied on me?" She flashed her eyes at him coldly. "What is his name," demanded Karl. "Who is he?" Then he hesitated for a moment. "No, I don't want to know." He got up slowly, took his coat and the bag he had already packed, and left the apartment. He could stay with Peter for a while. He needed some time.

Two days later, he received a big envelope. Ilona had sent him the photos. And she had written him a letter. It gave him a chill when he read it. He couldn't believe she would do such a thing to him. She was very detailed in portraying the guy, their nights together, and the sex; she painted a glowing picture of him and raved about his talents. Bewildered, he put down the letter. Then he fetched the whiskey bottle from Peter's bar.

"Forget her. I told you that she is a bitch!" Peter had already had too much alcohol. His voice sounded a little slurry. "She just wanted to benefit from your reputation and your money. She's not worth the trouble." He lifted his glass again. Karl didn't answer. After a while he said, "Maybe. But that doesn't help. And that she is taking off with this young stud doesn't make it easier either." Then he was quiet. He couldn't and wouldn't talk about it. He was too confused. He felt as though he was standing beside himself.

Months passed without Karl reaching a solution. He didn't know what to do and how to go on. He lived from one day to the next. Meanwhile, he had found a new apartment, so that he wouldn't put strain on his friendship with Peter. Karl lived from day to day and pondered about his life. He had to find a goal. The only thing that distracted him was dragging pain above his heart every once in a while. But he hardly took notice of that either.

He tried in vain. He was unable to produce a single drop. He had noticed for quite some time now that he had problems. It took some time until the urine was flowing; often he had the feeling that he was unable to empty his bladder entirely. Sometimes the urinary stream became slower and weaker although

98

he wasn't finished. By now, he had to use the washroom all the time, but he just couldn't urinate more than just a fraction of the bladder content. He needed to go to the doctor. He hated to see the doctor. But his condition drove him crazy.

"It is the prostrate gland," the doctor told him. "Apparently, you have a tumor that prevents the urine from flowing off. You have to have surgery." The doctor looked at him, frowning. "I have to tell you that the surgery will influence your virility. It is almost certain that you won't be able to have sex any more." Then he looked into Karl's file. "Maybe that won't bother you as much, you are already 62 after all."

Karl felt his anger rising. This young snot nose had just castrated him verbally and declared that he didn't need sex any more. He looked at the doctor. Just finished university, Karl thought. He was still an intern, about 30 years old at most. Only a little older than the stud.

"You have to sign here and give your consent. I can then schedule your surgery for tomorrow if you like," the doctor explained to him. Karl shook his head. "Absolutely not. Have a nice day." He turned around and left the dumbfounded doctor standing there.

"I know a good urologist. He is still old school and tries treatments that don't involve surgery first," Peter said while he was already dialing the number. After a short conversation, he hung up. "You have an appointment tomorrow morning. I am sure he can help you."

They had attached a tube to drain the urine. His bladder was completely filled. "High time," the doctor had mumbled. Then he explained to Karl how to use the tube and had sent him home. "We will watch it. If it gets worse, you have to come back immediately."

"Why are you spending so much time with Eva these days? She is almost as young as Ilona." Peter shook his head. He seemed to be really angry. "I am not doing anything," Karl responded. "She called and wanted to go for a coffee. I liked the idea and agreed. She is a very nice person."

"Nice?" Peter bristled with anger. "She is Ilona's friend and is probably as eager to get her hands on your money as Ilona is. I am sure there is something behind it." Karl bent his head. "Theoretically, that's possible, but I doubt it. The two of them haven't seen each other for quite some time. And she knows that I will get a divorce, so she also knows that I will be broke. But there is nothing going on, anyway. I already said that." Peter waved aside Karl's reasoning. "You and your women. You never seem to smarten up. Incidentally, you have a problem right now." Almost gloatingly, he pointed to Karl's lower abdomen. "First you have to take care of that."

Karl hadn't felt that good for quite some time. Exhilarated, he went home. The doctor didn't find any changes regarding his condition, but it wasn't getting worse either. The flirt with Eva took his mind off his problems. The young woman really seemed to adore him. And today she had kissed him goodbye. They both had blushed like teenagers.

The phone rang. Before Karl could even say his name, he heard Ilona's voice. "Hello sweetheart. Why don't we just forget what happened and you move back home," she purred. Karl swallowed hard. "What do you mean? I am supposed to forget that you sleep around with other guys and are obviously happier doing that than being with me? Didn't you write in your letter that I can't keep up with your new friend? What is this sudden change of mind about? I don't want you any more." "YOU don't want me any more?" She screamed into the receiver. "But you want Eva, right? I am no longer good enough for you, and now you try to seduce my friend, is that it? You pig, you womanizer, you...." Slowly, Karl put down the receiver. He couldn't believe what he just heard.

"Of course, she's jealous. She suddenly realizes what a good person you are." For half an hour already Peter had been busy analyzing Karl and his affairs with women, as he called it. Karl didn't listen very carefully. He was watching a thriller on TV. Eva had called in the afternoon. She had been beside herself; she had apologized and told him that she didn't know what was wrong with Ilona. "She called me and screamed at me that I should keep my hands off you. I have no idea what that was about. I certainly don't want to interfere with your relationship." She sounded as though she was almost crying. "Obviously, she and her boyfriend broke up. She said that, apparently, he had their photos taken and sent them to you. However, I can't imagine what he thought he might gain from that." He had calmed Eva down and arranged a date for the next day. He needed to think about everything. It took a few weeks before he had made up his mind.

He felt a searing pain in the left half of his body. It shot through the arm into his chest and took his breath away. "That's it," he thought and touched his breast. "I am having a heart attack. That's the last thing I needed. He breathed quickly to alleviate the pain a little bit. After five minutes he started to feel better, and ten minutes later he could breathe freely again. He was relieved and dismissed the incident, thinking, "Probably false alarm, I was lucky." Then he fell asleep.

Things were going better, including his urine flow problem. Karl whistled on his way to the doctor who confirmed Karl's impression. "It looks good. It seems that you don't need surgery after all."

Then he looked at Karl with a questioning expression on his face. "You certainly have the disposition of an elephant. How can you be so sure?" Karl shrugged his shoulders. "I am not sure that it will disappear again. But the attitude of one of your colleagues, who was sure it wouldn't get better, made me think." With these words he left the doctor's office. Eva was waiting for him.

"Your new apartment is really nice." Eva snuggled up to him. "You have good taste." "I know," Karl grinned and kissed her. "Ilona was furious when she heard about our relationship. But I don't care. After all, she didn't want you any more." She snuggled up to him even closer, pulling the blanket closer around both of them. "I didn't expect to find myself in bed with you so quickly." "Quickly?" Karl lifted his fingers and counted. "You call three months quick? Actually, it was more of a waiting game." Eva started to chuckle. "But it was worth it."

Conflict and Resolution

Karl suffered a nasty genital conflict when his considerably younger wife had sex with an equally young man, and he learned about her betrayal in a brutal way through the photos. In the conflict active phase, a prostate carcinoma grew, which partly compressed the urethra, so that the urine could no longer flow off.

The conflict was resolved when an equally young woman showed an honest interest in him and his wife became jealous. From this moment on, the tumor was decomposed and the urine could flow again. The traditional therapy had included prostrate laser surgery, which probably would have left him impotent.

Often, the person involved doesn't even notice that he has a prostate tumor, because it neither hurts nor causes other problems. Many patients see the doctor only after the tumor is gone, because they feel tired and weak. There are only few cases where the tumor compresses the urethra completely and, therefore, is noticed.

Karl's conflict is very clear. In many cases, however, the conflict can't be linked so obviously to a girlfriend or wife. Often, it is enough for a man to be "hit below the belt" or to be "degraded" in his job, for example. Representative conflicts also occur quite often, where men experience such a conflict in place of friends, fathers, or sons.

But the nasty genital conflict was not the only conflict Karl suffered. In addition, he experienced a conflict of territory loss. During the conflict active phase, small necroses developed in the coronary arteries. Karl noticed the effects in the form of angina pectoris, that is, dragging pain above the heart. When Karl met another woman the conflict was resolved. The epileptoid crisis manifested itself in a small heart attack a few weeks later.

The Punching Bag

• Jörg and the pleura

"Come on, give up. Say that it's enough." The big, heavy boy gasped. He was breathing heavily, his forehead was sweaty, and his face distorted. Again he yelled violently at the smaller boy he had in a headlock. He kept boxing his chest. Over and over again, like a robot. The blows sounded dull. The younger boy was obviously hurt by this attack against his left chest. But he clenched his teeth. He tenaciously refused to give up. In between, he uttered, "You can keep on hitting, but you won't break me."

He was probably 13 years old, small but wiry. His attacker was at least three years older. And he seemed increasingly desperate. Furiously, he took the head of the smaller boy between his hands, hit it on hard ground and continued to beat him, always with the right fist to the side of the heart. He became more and more furious. "I beat you to death," he yelled. He almost cried while he repeated it several times. For ten minutes he kept up the wild beating before he suddenly let go of his victim, pushed him away, and snarled, "Don't you dare to tell on me. That was just the beginning." With these words he stomped away towards the house, heavily breathing.

Jörg stayed down breathlessly. He knew he'd won. Without one single blow he had defeated his cousin. He had endured the brutal beating tenaciously and without turning a hair. But every fiber of his body had exuded his contempt for Matthias. Every punch that hit his skinny body had said, "You can't do anything to me. You are too weak." And Matthias had felt it. Definitely.

Jörg concealed the pain. He looked dirty and tousled and he tried to breathe very carefully. The pain went through his chest like a wave. It recurred again and again.

"What on earth happened to you?" His grandmother stared at him angrily and looked over him. "Where have you been? Why is your shirt so dirty? And your pants have a hole. Accusingly, she pointed to the waistband, which was in fact torn. Jörg didn't even try to give an excuse. He knew from experience that his grandmother wouldn't listen to him. He would have to fix his pants himself anyway.

He walked past Matthias and glanced at him. Matthias stared to the ground. When Jörg had almost passed him, he looked up. And he looked directly into the smiling face of his victim. He turned red immediately, bit his lips, and bolted out of the room.

"Yes," Jörg decided, "I won. He won't touch me ever again." Satisfied, he went to his small room behind the kitchen to change his clothes.

Jörg didn't mention the incident to anyone. Who should he talk to anyway? His grandmother, who cared for him and his two cousins, wasn't interested in these things. He saw his mother only on the weekends and he would have preferred to avoid these encounters. Presumably, so would she. The only person he could talk to was his grandfather. But that would look like he was telling on Matthias. So he didn't mention it. It wasn't important. In fact, he had forgotten the reason for the violent attack. It wasn't of interest any longer.

With his second cousin, Jan, he got along well. Jan was an intelligent boy, 17 years old, and not a bit arrogant. Sometimes he took Jörg to his friends. Nobody had a problem with that; they soon became his pals as well. Matthias didn't belong to this group. "Hey, you have to win tomorrow," one of the boys said and padded Jörg on the shoulder. He winced briefly. Then he listened inside himself. The pain was mostly gone. After all, it had been three weeks since Matthias had beaten him up. And meanwhile, the bruises had also turned yellow. Buoyantly, he grinned at the boy, "No problem. We are better soccer players."

Nervously, the doctor ran onto the playing field; the boys from the team were standing around Jörg in confusion. He realized it, but everything seemed shrouded in fog. He couldn't go on. Just like that, in the middle of the game. He couldn't breathe any more. "I'm OK," he murmured. But the doctor forced him to sit down on the floor." "You stay right where you are. You have to go to the hospital. We have to examine you a little closer," he decided. The game was over for Jörg.

"We diagnosed TB and an inflammation of the pleura," the doctor explained to Jörg's mother. "He definitely has to stay in the hospital. We will treat him with antibiotics and then we'll see how things progress." With these words, he let her go to see her son.

"Damn." Jörg was awake. Still. The doctors had told him that he had a prolonged treatment in front of him, which meant that he could forget about soccer for the time being. He didn't know how things would go from there. That's what his mother has told him laconically. Jörg couldn't help but realize her indifference. But he was used to it, it didn't matter to him any more. What did matter to him, though, was the fact that he had to stay in the hospital.

The doctor raised his eyebrow when he looked at the X-ray. "A pleural effusion developed. A lot of fluid has accumulated in the chest. We will have to get the fluid out with a cannula," he said. Then he turned directly to Jörg. "That won't be fun, buddy, but we need to do it."

Jörg sighed. For days he has been in the hospital without any change of his condition. They gave him all kinds of pills and drops, but the result was always the same worried frowning of the doctor. At any rate, they suddenly found out that he didn't have TB after all. They couldn't find anything any more. "The intern's mistake," the head physician had decided.

They had aspirated fluid from his chest three times already. Every time, it was a terrible ordeal. Afterwards, his condition would improve temporarily, but then fluid would build up again. But Jörg was most concerned about the doctors' increasing helplessness.

When his grandfather visited him, he vented his feelings. "Grandpa, please get me out of here. I am not getting better, they can't help me," he begged and looked at the old man. "I will only get sicker." His grandfather was very worried, but he nodded and said, "I will convince your mother to have you released from the hospital. I promise."

His grandfather kept his promise. Jörg didn't have any idea how he convinced his mother to sign the consent form to have Jörg released despite the hue and cry of the doctors.

"You will kill him," the head physician shouted angrily. "Don't be so stubborn. If necessary, I have to get a warrant. Do you know that the court can revoke custody from you if you inflict harm on your child? The doctor became more and more angry and agitated the more stoic his mother was. Jörg had to grin to himself. "Revoking custody surely would make her day," he thought and his grin became even broader. His mother didn't care at all about what the doctor said. And neither did she care about him.

It was getting better.
With every passing day Jörg could breathe easier, his arm, which was almost immobile, and his entire shoulder, which was tense, became more relaxed. He didn't take the drugs any longer. He had flushed them down the toilet immediately after he had returned home. As long as he couldn't go to school, he spent a lot of time with his grandfather in the garden. His grandfather taught him a lot of things about plants and animals. Jörg wasn't particularly interested in these things, but he loved his grandfather's warm, deep voice. And since he had got him out of the hospital, he loved him even more. Sometimes, Jörg took his grandfather's callous hand into his own hand. Just like that.

"Come on, Jörg, score a goal! Come on!" The spectators yelled full of excitement. They cheered him on during his sprint towards the other team's net. He was running alone, no offside. A dream situation. Then he saw the anxious face of the goaltender. He was a boy, maybe 13 years old, who knew that he barely had a chance. Jörg grinned at him, put the ball in the right position while he was running and put the ball above the goalie's shoulder directly into the net. "Score, score!" the fans shouted. The final whistle sounded; Jörg's team was the new youth champion. Ecstatically, the boys of his team carried Jörg on their shoulders, everybody was screaming and more and more people came running to congratulate them. Jörg cheered the loudest. Then he saw a face at the edge of the playing field. Matthias immediately looked into the other direction. He turned around quickly and disappeared in the crowd. Jörg sent a thunderous cheer in his direction. "Victory!!!!"

Conflict and Resolution

During the fight with his cousin, Jörg suffered a biological conflict of an attack against the inner chest. Afterwards, cell multiplication at the left pleura took place. However, Jörg noticed the cell multiplication only when it was in the healing phase – through the cell decomposition and the accompanying healing edema.

He had shortness of breath and the doctors in the hospital diagnosed an inflammation of the pleura and, in addition, the existence of TB-like bacteria. They decompose tumors or other additional tissue. A pleural effusion occurs during the healing phase through the fluid that develops during the decomposition.

Because of the constant draining of the fluid and the ordeal connected to it, Jörg was set on a real track. The conflict relapsed. He experienced an attack against the inner chest over and over again. Only by leaving the hospital was Jörg able to let his body heal without interferences.

Nobody Is Calling Me...

• Nina and the suicide

Do I want to have breakfast or not? Nina asked herself. Actually, she wasn't hungry at all. She attributed it to her age that she was already awake. "You just don't need as much sleep," she thought and looked at the clock. It was only 5:30 a.m. on a day she didn't like anyway. Now it would be endlessly long besides everything else.

A Saturday. It already looked a lot like fall, although summer wasn't over yet. "At least that's what the calendar says," she corrected herself. In fact, summer was mostly over at this time of year. "It's September after all. Neither fish nor fowl," she thought, a little melancholic.

Lost in thought, she picked up the coffee pot. She actually didn't like this brew any longer. It had been different when Tim had brought her coffee in bed. She had enjoyed every sip. Quickly, she dismissed the thought. It wasn't good for her to think about Tim. Then she became sad, sadder than she already was anyway. She never would have thought to survive him for so many years. She missed him very much. Being close to him, his tenderness, even the sex they had. Who said that you had to be young to enjoy sex. At any rate, Nina missed Tim also physically.

She remembered the time when she had just met Tim. He was always busy. They rarely saw each other. But that made their time together special. She waited entire evenings for his calls, for his voice that would whisper into her ear how much he loved her. Or would tell her that he was coming by. Nina sighed. She would never forget the day when he called and said he needed time for himself. "Nina, I met someone else. I don't know what to think about this. I need time to make up my mind." It still gave her a chill. At that time she had been waiting for three days to hear from him. And then he told her something like that. She was devastated.

She had experienced something similar before with her first boyfriend. Apart from kissing and petting nothing serious happened. At that time, she had been just 16 and she was so much in love. Until that evening. They hadn't actually arranged for a date, but she wanted to tell him something very quickly before going home. She couldn't find him anywhere. He wasn't in the yard and his parents didn't know where he was either. Finally, she had heard voices in the barn. She walked in and found the two of them. He was lying half-naked in the arms of a girl she knew by sight. The girl was much older than him and Nina. But that's what obviously attracted him. After that experience, Nina fell into depression.

In the end, Tim had decided to stay with her. They got married and had two sons. But sometimes she doubted that he really had to be in the office that long. He smelled differently too, seemed absent-minded, and criticized her. Nina didn't want to see it. She didn't want to know what he did and whom he did it with. "I was a coward," she admitted to herself. "I should have dealt with it. I suppressed the problem instead, but I could never really forget it."

Lost in thought, she wiped the kitchen table. Then she put the coffee pot back. "A glass of milk will be enough," she decided. She walked over to the phone while she sipped her milk. Her sons had been telling her for quite some

106

time that she needed a new one. Sometimes it made a noise and the receiver would get caught in the storage dish. She assumed it was a manufacturing error. Someone miscalculated and the earpiece and the storage dish didn't fit ever since. She picked up the receiver and held it against her ear. "Beep, beep," sounded the free line signal. She shook her head and hung up again. "I am silly. At this time none of the boys will be up yet. They will call at about 9:00 a.m. at the earliest."

Then she smiled a little melancholically. Well, the boys weren't boys any longer. They were grown men now. Lukas, her older son, lived with his wife in a way she would have never wished for herself. No, she wouldn't interfere. But still, sometimes she wished for him to be more self-confident and end this drama. Her grandson would be able to deal with a separation better than with the current situation.

Nina picked up the remote control and started zapping through the channels. She couldn't find anything interesting to watch. Again, she looked first at the phone and then to the clock. It was 6:50 a.m. Suddenly she got up, grabbed her coat, put on her comfortable shoes, and left the apartment. Outside, she looked around. "The day isn't bad at all," she decided. It had been raining during the night. The street seemed fresh. The leaves that were still clinging to the trees exude something new. Thick clouds still crowded in the sky, but they would disappear soon. Here and there you could already see a piece of blue sky. Determinedly, she started walking.

She crossed the street in front of the house, nodded to her neighbour at the bakery, and kept on walking determinedly. Mrs. Berg was a gossip. And she had already had this nosy look on her face. She was all Nina needed right now. There was only one thing to do: Don't give her a chance.

Ten meters further a man ran into her. "What's with you, old hag? Watch where you're goin'!" he grumbled. She turned around angrily. "You better be careful that I don't kick you you know where, you idiot," she railed. The man turned around with a surprised expression on his face, but he didn't say anything. "That came certainly unexpected for this guy," she thought, satisfied with herself. Then she blushed a little. "I was pretty vulgar," she admitted to herself. But it had been fun nonetheless. "And that's what counts, right?" She didn't get a response. A young woman just gave her a strange look while she was passing. That was OK. Nina shrugged her shoulders.

Two and a half hours later she unlocked her apartment door. Circumstantially, she pulled her shoes from her feet. That wasn't as easy, because her feet were swollen from the long walk. The shoes just didn't want to come off. A little exhausted, she hung her coat; then she looked at the clock. It was 8:50 a.m. Mechanically, she went over to the phone and stared at the answering machine. No blinking. Nobody had called. "It is still to early, don't get worked up," she scolded herself. Then she checked the machine. It worked. She turned around and sat down on the couch. She picked up her book; she still loved to read.

Just when Nina had managed to delve into her book – the paragraph was suspenseful, even if she knew Stephen King almost by heart by now – the doorbell rang. She looked up in astonishment. It was 9:30 a.m. She knew for sure that it couldn't be her sons. If any, they had probably just got up and were taking a shower. The mail? Hardly. The phone was much more convenient than writing letters.

She rose with an effort. Her back was hurting. Gradually, she could feel the years catching up. When she opened the door, her neighbour beamed at her. "Happy birthday, Mrs. Rossi. Today is your birthday, right? I brought you something." And with that, she handed Nina a cake and a few mingy sunflowers and squeezed through the door into the apartment. She looked around curiously. "So? Has the family already called?" Her look became almost greedy when she asked the question. Then she spun around the room. She realized the lack of flowers and cards. She turned to Nina again and beamed at her. "But it is still early in the morning. I wanted to say happy birthday earlier, but you went by the bakery so fast and then it was my turn. So, I thought I'd just come by. I have to say, you are in pretty good shape considering your age." She enviously looked over Nina. Nina turned around. She didn't want to be impolite today. But at the same time, a sarcastic remark was on the tip of her tongue. However, she controlled herself.

She looked at her neighbour with a constrained smile. "That is really nice of you. But I have do make some preparations. My children have invited me for lunch. We are going to the Pittaccia. I would like to apply a facial mask and do my nails. So I just have half an hour. Would you like a cappuccino?" "Oh, yes, I would love to." Mrs. Berg didn't seem to notice that she wasn't welcome.

She passed Nina, hurried into the living room and broke into ecstasy. "How nicely you arranged this room. And so comfortable."

Without asking, she fell into Tim's favourite chair. Nina was about to go to the kitchen, but when she saw this gossiping, disagreeable hag sitting in Tim's chair she couldn't control herself any longer. "Get up," she hissed. "Pardon me?" Mrs. Berg was confused. "Leave, now. I don't want to see or to hear you. And take your stupid cake and this poor excuse of a bunch of flowers. Get out!"

Her eyes flashed very angrily. Nina appeared to be almost ten centimeters taller than before. Stammering, her neighbour got up. "But, but…."

"Get out," Nina hissed one last time and held the door open. Mrs. Berg quickly grabbed her presents and almost ran out of the apartment. She collected herself only when she had reached the hallway. While Nina slammed the door, she started bickering. "Old hag! I just wanted to give her a little joy and now this. She can't treat me like that. Just because nobody cares any more…. That's not my fault…."

It kept resonating for a while. Nina leaned against the wall with her eyes closed. Was her neighbour right? Was that the way she behaved? Maybe a little, she admitted to herself. Sometimes she was very depressed. However, that was not because of her children. She grieved for Tim. It had already been ten years that he had dropped dead from a heart attack. Nothing unusual considering his age; she knew that. Tim had been 75. But she wasn't interested in what was unusual or not. She wanted him. Without him, life wasn't fun any longer. "For him to die on my birthday must have been his dark humour," Nina thought. Today, she turned 75. Not that old, as everybody affirmed her over and over again. But sometimes she felt as though she was already dead.

108

"Why aren't the boys calling," she suddenly asked herself and looked at the clock. It was almost 10:00 a.m. That was unusual. They would always call. And in the afternoon they would come over for a coffee with their families and stay for dinner.

Since her older son had these marital problems, she didn't enjoy it as much, but on the other hand, she liked the swarming activity around her. "Was there some truth in what Mrs. Berg had said? Am I just a burden for them? Do they still like their mother?" she suddenly asked herself. Could it be possible that her gossiping, nosy neighbour was right? "No," Nina decided and went back to her couch. Absent-mindedly, she tried to concentrate on her book again.

It was 1:00 p.m. and nobody had called yet. She hadn't received any birthday greeting and didn't know whether they would still come over for coffee at around 4:00 p.m. That was the time they had agreed on, because they had to comply with her youngest grandson's need for a nap. He was only two years old, a late arrival. If he didn't get enough sleep, he would be very fussy.

She looked at the clock again. The hand had moved to 1:05 p.m. She put the book aside, walked over to the phone, and stared at it. "Ring! Come on. Right now." But the telephone didn't do anything. It didn't make a sound. Irresolutely, she looked to the clock again. It was 1:07 p.m.
I am taking a bath now," she decided. She had lied about going out to the restaurant and, therefore, there was no need to get dolled up. But she liked to have a bath. Still. And she had time; she had all the time in the world.

She startled up. She had almost fallen asleep. The clock said 2:13 p.m. Did she miss the ringing of the phone? She got out of the tub quickly. A little bit too quickly, because everything went black. "I shouldn't do that," she thought, "it could be dangerous." She was drying herself off when she suddenly stopped. "Actually, why shouldn't I?"

They found her at 4:30 p.m. She was lying in the tub, half-dressed. Her sons looked at her in disbelief. Her daughters in law quickly took the children and left the apartment. They cried when they took them to the playground in front of the house, so that the children wouldn't see her dead grandmother. While the doctor issued the death certificate, – drowned after taking sleeping pills – her sons read her last note. "I know that there is nothing left to do for me here. You don't miss me, and that's how it is supposed to be. I want to be with Tim again. For Lukas: Give yourself and your wife a chance and separate." Below was another P.S. "At least you could have called. I was waiting the whole time."

Both men – one was chunky with a slight belly and beginning to get bald; the other was tall, almost gangling, with grey strands in his dark hair and wearing glasses – looked surprised at each other with their eyes full of tears. "I tried at least ten times to reach her. The line was busy all the time," the tall man said. "Me too," the smaller one responded. "I thought she was drowning in birthday calls.
At this moment, they heard the babbling of a child in the hallway. Robert, Lukas's son obviously escaped from his mother and the doctor hadn't closed the apartment door properly. Now he wobbled on his little, chunky legs into the apartment. Waving cheerfully, he disappeared into the living room. Both men ran after him. Lukas cursed, "Can't she at least watch the kid?"

Then he caught his son who was about to climb onto the couch. Robert nudged Lukas's face with his small, chunky index finger in. "Daddy crying? Has an ouch?" he asked with an astonished expression on his face. Lukas turned his head to the side and wiped the tears from his face. Then he looked at his brother.

He was standing there like a statue. He stared at the phone. "What's the matter, Benni?" Lukas asked. He was curious and came closer. Even Robert looked attentively in the direction of the spot his uncle was staring at. And then they saw it: The receiver was stuck.

Conflict and Resolution

Nina suffered a female sexual conflict with her first love when her boyfriend betrayed her. Being a left-handed woman, that caused her depression. It is possible that she also had dragging pain above the heart, angina pectoris.

When she suffered a sexual conflict again with Tim, her future husband, who also had an affair with another woman, the depression was resolved and Nina entered a so-called post-mortal constellation. Whenever she hit the track "Does he really love me? Am I still important to him?" in the future, for example, when she assumed that her husband had another affair, she became manic and considered suicide.

In left-handed women, the post-mortal constellation consists of conflict 1, which is a female sexual conflict, and conflict 2, another female sexual conflict. In right-handed women, conflict 1 would be a female sexual conflict and conflict 2 a loss of territory conflict.

Three aspects were part of her track on her birthday: the grief for Tim, who had died on her birthday; the question whether she was loved and needed at all, in this case by her sons; and the waiting at the phone, which she had done so often in the past.

Every time she had to wait for Tim's call, she hit the track. It continued even after his death, whenever she had the feeling that she wasn't loved because the other person didn't call, so that Nina entered a suicidal constellation. In the end, she committed suicide.

The Loss
• Lukas and testicular cancer

"How could she do that? How could she do that to us? She just had to know that we would come over for coffee and find her." Lukas racked his brains. He didn't understand his mother. As if it wasn't enough that she died unexpected, no, she had committed suicide. Just because of a broken phone. At least, that's how it appeared to Lukas.

He still felt like being in a different world. Meanwhile, three months had passed. Months, during which Lukas barely got hardly any sleep and had lost ten kilos. He couldn't talk to anybody about his worries. Benni had many friends. Lukas was on his own most of the time. There was no way he could talk to his wife about these things. For months, they had lived separate lives. He had to admit to himself that Robert was the only reason they were still together.

For several days he had been experiencing dragging pain in his right testicle. It was not bad enough, though, to do something. He didn't really worry just yet. However, he noticed it in his sub-conscience. It was a minor matter.

Lukas had made up his mind. He would confront her. She couldn't just do a vanishing trick and leave him with his questions, self-doubts, and self-reproaches. Determinedly, he strode towards the cemetery, which was close by. He felt it was time for a nice winter walk. It was shortly before Christmas, the right time to resolve the situation.

Lukas stared at his parent's grave. At first, he was just talking in his thoughts. Then, he started voicing his thoughts. He didn't notice that some of the mourners were watching him; some were startled, others confused, and others again wondering or understanding.

Lukas was talking to his parents. He told them about the time when he had done that test of courage with Benni and both of them had fallen into the basement of the ruins of the old industrial building. They couldn't get out until Lukas had constructed some kind of a ladder from rusted iron girders, which they used to climb out. "I thought that there were ghosts or something in there," Lukas recounted. "We were very scared. Nobody would have heard or found us."

Lost in thought, Lukas looked at the ivy. Benni and Lukas had vowed never to tell anyone and they had kept their oath. "Until today," Lukas said. "But that's OK. Benni will understand." Only once, Benni wanted to tell something. That was when Lukas had developed laryngitis after their adventure. But his brother's warning look had prevented him for doing so.

Then he remembered his wedding. "Dad, you advised against it. But I didn't understand you. How could you think I would listen to you?" Lukas shook his head. "But you were right. My wife and I are just too different. It won't work out in the long run."

Now he had a smile on his face. "Do you remember, mom, how Robert looked when he was born? He looked a little bit like dad. Full of wrinkles, alert, with the typical prominent ears." Lukas laughed. Again, the people visiting the cemetery glanced at him. He didn't care. "Now, both of you are gone, we lost you. That isn't easy."

His voice became lower and lower. At first, he didn't realize that he was crying. Only when he was mechanically looking for a tissue in his pocket did he become aware of it. He didn't care. The crying felt good. People could think what they wanted. Lukas was mourning the loss of his parents.

He was outside in the cold for two hours. Meanwhile, it had started to snow. "Robert will be thrilled," thought Lukas. "A white Christmas. When was the last time we had that," he seemed to ask his parents. Eventually, he turned around. "Bye," he murmured towards the grave before he tramped home through the snow.

He was scared when he examined his testicle. He could feel a lump in the spot where the other testicle was soft. He would have to have that examined by a doctor. For now, he wouldn't tell his wife anything about it.

"I strongly recommend surgery," the doctor said after the examination. "It appears to be testicular cancer. It will be best if we remove the testicle in order to make sure that we prevent metastases. You are still young. Your chances of healing are good."

Lukas was dumbfounded. Why were all these things happening to him? And if that wasn't enough, everything happened at the same time. Now he might die from testicular cancer. Bewildered, he went home. That evening, he finally talked to his wife like they hadn't been talking in a long time. And she, as well, talked to him about other things than just Robert's problems in the kindergarten. Both of them seemed like frightened children.

They both had made a decision. Lukas wouldn't undergo surgery. He had plainly refused it. His wife couldn't convince him otherwise. When she realized that her attempts were futile, she gave up. "I will support you, no matter what you decide," she had said.

Lukas's decision had a great deal to do with fear. Fear of the hospital, fear of soulless doctors, stressed nurses, suffering people, and sad faces. Lukas would never admit it, but his fear of the hospital was bigger than his fear of cancer. So, he just waited.

The lump hadn't grown any more. Every day, Lukas had felt it and was relieved when he found that it had remained the same size. He had hardly any pain. His fear lay beyond the surface. Sometimes he had the feeling that his fear had disappeared. He couldn't explain why he was so certain all of a sudden.

The whole situation had already resulted in one good thing. His marriage had never been as good as it was now. He and his wife seemed to really get along for the first time. They had come close. Winter was over; spring was here. A new beginning was in front of them.

"Strange. Are sure you don't want to have surgery?" The doctor looked at Lukas suspiciously. "Yes, I am sure," was Lukas's answer. "I don't have any problems." Helplessly, the doctor scratched his head. "Well, it is your decision." Then he shook his hand and said goodbye.

"Can I come, daddy?" Robert still looked a little dozily. He had just woken up from his nap. "OK, but we have to hurry." Lukas grinned at his little son. Robert ran to get his pants, put them on the wrong way, fell down, and snorted with laughter. Lukas had to laugh as well. Then he helped Robert to get dressed.

"Do you think grandma and grandpa can hear us?" Robert stood in front of his grandparents' grave. "Certainly," Lukas responded. "I told them so many things and it would be senseless if they didn't hear it, right?" Robert nodded. "What did they say? Do you think they would talk to me as well?" "They don't talk like we talk. You can hear their answers inside you. Sometimes, they also talk through messengers.

Lukas would find himself between the devil and the deep blue sea if he continued like this. What was he thinking mentioning messengers? That was monkey business. He was putting weird ideas in Robert's head. "Like this one?" Robert held up a ladybug. "Maybe." Lukas appeared only little relieved.

"What does it tell you?" he asked carefully. "That they love us," responded Robert. "And mom as well." Then he twinkled mischievously at his father. "And my sister as well."

"What sister?" Lukas frowned. "Well, the one that I will have. Because I wished for it." Robert looked very important. "I will protect her and teach her how to ride the scooter and play Cowboys and Indians with her."

"You will, won't you, hmm?" Lukas took his son's hand in his. Robert had many more ideas of what he would do with his sister. Lukas didn't really listen any more. He thought for a while; then he decided that it wasn't such a bad idea at all. He was curious what his wife would think of Robert's idea.

Conflict and Resolution

Lukas suffered a severe conflict of loss when his mother committed suicide. During the conflict active phase, tissue necroses occurred in the right testicle (mother-child side for left-handed people), which he hardly felt except for a mild twinge. His visit to the cemetery and his intensive conversation with his parents resolved the conflict; he entered the healing phase. As a consequence, a cyst developed and the testicle swelled. The doctor diagnosed testicle cancer.

The testicular cyst has the biological meaning to produce more testosterone to balance the suffered loss. Lukas's brother, Benni, has also suffered a loss; however, he didn't develop a DHS. That doesn't mean that their mother's death was a less shocking experience for him. But obviously, not all three preconditions for a DHS coincided, so that he didn't have to go through testicle cancer or another Special Biological Program.

Another conflict from Lukas's childhood is briefly mentioned. He suffered a fear-due-to-shock conflict, when he and his brother fell into the basement of the old industrial building and he thought they were going to die there. During the healing phase, he developed laryngitis.

The Affair
• Felix and multiple sclerosis

The shock went through Felix like cold lightning. His heart almost stopped beating and he stared to the other side of the street. Yes, it was Dietmar, a very good colleague of his wife. Britta got along with him very well; she talked to him pretty much about everything, so that sometimes, Felix had become jealous of their close relationship and their feelings for each other. Dietmar was the last thing he needed right now. He quickly stopped in front of a store window, dragged Linda with him, and pretended to be interested in the window display. Dietmar was reflected in the window pane. "He saw me," it went through Felix's head. "Clearly, he also recognized me." He feverishly tried to decide what he should do now. He saw Dietmar hesitating. A few minutes ago he had wanted to cross the street and say hello to Felix. Now, he turned, shrugged his shoulders, and kept on walking on his side of the street.

"Sweetheart, are you interested in esoterism?" Linda's voice jolted Felix out of his thoughts. "What?" He looked at her questioningly; then he glanced at the window display. A motley collection of strange stones and boxes, books, the titles of which promised "What You Want To Know About Basic Chakra," and necklaces, dream catchers, and incense lay and hung in the window more or less randomly. Felix frowned. "Let's keep going." Lost in thoughts, he walked ahead, while Linda was following him, puzzled.

Linda had attracted his attention last night at the bar in the hotel. Felix wasn't actually a person to visit bars, least of all during a business trip when he had to stay in a hotel. Neither did he like one-night stands. He had never had one. And yet, that's exactly what happened.

First he had visited the bar, then he had met Linda, who was on a business trip as well, and, eventually, they had ended up in bed. The fact that Linda was still with him the next day showed how inexperienced he was in these matters. Obviously, she had expected more. And he hadn't had the courage to end it right there.

"Now I'm in trouble," Felix thought. Dietmar had seen him hand in hand with another woman. And Linda had probably kissed him that very moment. She had constantly clung to him. Dietmar would tell Britta, no doubt. And Britta would divorce him. Felix didn't have any doubts about that either. "And you don't deserve any better, you idiot," he said to himself. "To jeopardize everything for Linda, a woman you met in a bar. Man oh man...."

"Hi, honey." Felix gave Britta a kiss. She hugged him impartially and kissed him back. "How was your trip? You look exhausted." With these words she helped him take off his coat. Felix had never been so insecure. Did she know it already? It had been three days. Dietmar had had all the time in the world to tell her. Felix looked at her face inquiringly. No, apparently, Dietmar hadn't told her yet. Felix felt sick just thinking about it. Carefully, he stroked back her hair. Then he gave her a kiss on the cheek. "I missed you. Let's curl up on the couch and relax."

Three weeks later, Britta still appeared impartial. Felix caught himself watching her in anticipation of the disaster. Sometimes, he virtually wished for it to happen, so that the fear would go away. He could barely sleep; he

116

kept having the same dream. Britta was walking away from him and turned around once before she walked on. And then he saw Dietmar's face. He was laughing, he seemed to have a real fit of laughter. At this point, Felix usually woke up. The dream seemed so real.

"There is Bodo and Katrin, Melinda and Daniel, and, of course, Dietmar and Gerlinde. We want to barbeque and have a little campfire. That will be lots of fun. Britta was thrilled. And normally, Felix would look forward to it as well.

He and Britta mostly had the same friends. This time, however, he was scared. Dietmar would be there too. How should he behave towards him? Felix's thoughts were racing. He had to find an excuse for staying home. But if he didn't show up, wouldn't that awake Dietmar's attention more than ever and prompt him to ask about Felix? Maybe, he would then use the opportunity and the relaxed atmosphere to insinuate things. No, Felix couldn't take that risk. He would go, although it was difficult for him.

Felix became more and more insecure. Dietmar was as friendly as ever. He never mentioned their disastrous encounter during Felix's business trip. But Felix was unable to relax. All evening, he was waiting for the blow.

"What is the matter, Felix?" He could hear the resentment in Britta's voice. You are as tense as an examinee. Hey, it's us and we are all friends. Relax." Felix offered a strained smile. She was right. He was completely tense. It couldn't go on like this.

But it did go on. Week after week and month after month. Felix suppressed the problem as best he could, but it was constantly existent. Subliminally, he was still afraid that Dietmar would tell Britta about Linda. And he was even more afraid of Britta's reaction. There was no doubt she would leave him. But Felix didn't want to lose her. He still had that dream, however, not as frequently.

"It has already been half a year," it struck Felix. He had just entered an appointment for Monday when he realized that that day his one-night stand dated back half a year. When he thought about what had happened then, Felix felt sick. His heart beat faster and he had wobbly knees. He stared at the date in the calendar. Then he came to a conclusion. He would tell Britta the truth, no matter what would happen afterwards. It just couldn't go on like this.

"Why?" Britta looked at him in bewilderment. "I mean, why are you suddenly telling me about it after such a long time?" You have been absent-minded and nervous the whole time because of it? And was it worth it?" Felix looked at her unhappily. "I wish I hadn't done it. I was so stupid, I don't know why. I was so afraid that you'd leave me. That's why I didn't say anything." "And why did you do it now?" asked Britta. "I could have pretty well done without that information," she snapped at him. Pleadingly, he stretched out his hand to touch her, but she moved away from him immediately. "You might have heard it from someone else and that would have made things even worse."

Looking a picture of misery, he stood in the kitchen. He felt small. He looked tired and he had dark rings under his eyes. Felix had lost weight. He was slender to begin with, but now he appeared skinny. A feeling of tenderness came over Britta. She almost wanted to give him a hug. But another feeling kept her from doing it: disappointment, grief, and the feeling of betrayal. No matter what the two of them would do, nothing would be like it had been before. Felix had destroyed something.

Felix still couldn't believe how lucky he was. Britta hadn't left him. She hadn't even seriously considered it. Sure, she had been sad and also hurt, for a while she had been unable to bear being touched by him, and during the first few days she didn't want to talk to him about it. But meanwhile, their relationship started to normalize again. That was Felix's impression anyway.

It had been four weeks since Felix had confessed his affair to Britta. He only realized now how energy draining the situation had been. He felt tired, much more tired that usual. He was weak and feeble, yet relieved. Britta had forgiven him - more or less.

He rubbed his right eye, twinkled and squinted, but that didn't help. It felt as though he was looking through glasses with the right glass being masked. He could see with each eye only left from the middle. There was nothing next to it. He looked around, closed his eyes, opened them, but nothing changed. Nevertheless, he didn't want to see the doctor. He was getting ready to go to work. Britta hesitated to let him go, she was worried.

"What's the matter?" Udo started to get worried when he looked at Felix. Felix held his right arm, kneaded it and tried to move it. It was numb and he had pins and needles in his arm. Felix shrugged his left shoulder. "I don't know. It is numb all of a sudden. I can't feel it any more." He had a frightened expression on his face when he looked at Udo, who decided without further ado to call the doctor. "You have to have that checked."

The doctor examined Felix's brain scans. "I suspect multiple sclerosis," he said. He didn't seem to notice the effect of his words on Felix. Felix looked at the doctor; he was horrified. "Multiple sclerosis? How did I develop multiple sclerosis all of a sudden," he thought, bewildered. "Does that mean that I will end up in a wheelchair?" Felix was shocked. He got up from his chair as if in trance. He had to see Britta. That would change everything. He didn't want to become her nursing case.

Felix didn't want to look into the faces of the passers-by. They didn't look at him anyway. They were looking at Britta. And the expression in their faces was pity. They felt pity for the young woman who was pushing the wheelchair with her young husband. Felix couldn't bear it any longer. Full of bitterness, he stared in front of him.

"Hey, you two," sounded Dietmar's voice. He hugged Britta hello and shook Felix's hand. "You know, it has been quite some time since we had some fun. How about we have a barbeque on Friday? The others will be there as well. We will have a little campfire and such, I'm sure we will have fun again."

Britta agreed immediately and Felix nodded absent-mindedly. He wanted to go home. And he certainly wouldn't go to the barbeque. But he would tell Britta later. Suspiciously, he watched Dietmar, who said goodbye to Britta, hugging her again. Didn't he look a little too long into her eyes? And too intense as well? And why wasn't he actually with Gina any longer, Felix asked himself suddenly. That thought changed his mind. He would probably go to the barbeque after all. He was quite certain.

Conflict and Resolution

Multiple sclerosis as an independent "disease" doesn't exist. In most cases, beginning motor and sensory dysfunctions results in a multiple sclerosis diagnosis.

Felix's symptoms included the loss of the visual field and the numbness in his arm, both occurring on the partner side, which is the right side in right-handed people, as is generally known. When he had an affair and Dietmar saw him with the other woman, Felix suffered a conflict of fear breathing down his neck of a visual separation as well as a separation anxiety conflict, that is, he was afraid of losing his partner from his embrace.

For half a year, he had been afraid that his affair would come out and Britta would leave him. When he finally confessed everything, he resolved his conflicts. Britta didn't leave him, Felix entered the healing phase, and during the epileptoid crisis four weeks later he suffered visual field loss of the right half of the visual field (after the visual separation anxiety conflict). The next day, his arm became numb. When the doctor examined Felix's brain scan, he found alterations – mostly Hamer Foci –, which he associated with multiple sclerosis.

This diagnosis triggers a second conflict in almost every patient, the conflict of "being unable to walk any more." For, most people, just like Felix, think of the wheelchair and of being doomed to never be able to walk again.

As a result of this conflict, the legs become weaker. Every time that happens, the patients suffer a relapse. Their legs become even weaker, and this process continues until they actually need a wheelchair. It is a vicious circle, which, the longer it lasts, the harder it gets to interrupt.

People who know the New Medicine won't get into this vicious circle. Felix didn't know about it and neither did Britta. It can take years until the patients permanently depend on the wheelchair. In Felix's case it happened relatively fast.

In the Blink of an Eye
• Susanne and the cataract

It happened very quietly. Later, Susanne often asked herself why he hadn't screamed at all. Just a moment ago, both were there, and a minute later she couldn't see him anywhere. She saw him thrashing his arms around and staring at her, his eyes wide open with fear; then he was gone. Susanne stared at the spot where she had just seen her brother's head. She could barely move. The seven-year-old girl wasn't able to grasp the truth yet. Sven was gone. He was probably dead. He had drowned in front of her eyes just then.

It was only hours later that they found the girl, who was chilled to the bones, on the frozen lake. She was standing there, stunned, and stared at the hole in the ice. Susanne didn't dare to move. She didn't want the ice to break under her as well. And she didn't want to leave her twin brother. It had to be ice-cold in the water. At least, she wanted to stay close to him.

"Why didn't you do anything? Why didn't you get help? Maybe he could have been saved." Her mother repeated the sentences over and over again. Susanne looked at her helplessly. She remained silent. She saw her mother crying and her father was numb. But Sven was gone, and that hurt the most. What should she do without her brother?

Susanne didn't talk to anybody about that day. She avoided every situation that would remind her of it. She functioned like a little robot. Her parents were preoccupied with their own grief. Nobody paid attention to the girl. Sometimes, when she had to walk passed the lake, everything inside her clenched. Then she would start running and look in the other direction.

"Sven isn't gone, not really." Karl nodded confirmatively when he said that. Then he drew at his cigarette and tried to sit a little more comfortably on the hard park bench. "He is always with you. It's the same with my Mia. She is here."

"Here with us? Where?" Susanne looked at Karl disbelievingly. They had become friends during the past weeks. Often, she came to the park to be alone. At some point, they had started talking. "You can feel it. You can't see them, but you can feel them. If you concentrate, you can sometimes hear them talk or laugh. Sometimes, Mia scolds me because I have become such a bum." Karl laughed quietly. "But I don't take that too seriously. She knows that that's actually not important."

Karl was a bum, a homeless person, who had been unable to get a foothold again after the death of his wife. He had told her a little bit about himself. Susanne liked him. Sometimes he brought things for her: a big shell, a stone with a hole, a particularly beautiful feather or a knobbed piece of wood. Sometimes he gave her things, other times he just pointed them out to her, but he always told stories about them. Karl was the only person Susanne could talk to about everything. Even about Sven's death.

Now she was listening. She tried to hold her head on an angle and kept her eyes closed. She even stopped breathing, so that she wouldn't miss anything. A little cloud of Karl's cigarette smoke got into her nose. Susanne opened her eyes. She looked at Karl in disappointment. "I can't hear or feel anything. Neither Mia nor Sven. I can just smell your cigarette. Irascibly, she poked with her feet in the sand.

"You have to practice it. I couldn't do it at first either. But since I know that Mia is still with me, I can live again." Then he looked over to the girl. "What about your parents?"

Susanne shook her head. "I can see and hear them, but they are not really there. I think mom is still blaming me for what happened. But it wasn't my fault. And dad is busy and working all the time." Pensively, Karl looked at the branches of a tree that were spreading above them. "Maybe they'll come back. If not, you have to accept it. I will always be there for you." Susanne sighed and got up. "I have to go home now. It is late." Karl nodded goodbye. "You have to practice, Susanne, then you will feel him. Believe me."

Susanne stared with open eyes into the dark. Again, she couldn't sleep. So she practiced. She concentrated very hard, but the only thing she could hear was the streetcar in front of the house. It just wouldn't work.

Susanne startled. She had heard something. A voice. The voice of a boy. Maybe Sven? Her heart was pounding. She was about to doze off when she heard it. Now it was gone again. Maybe that's what Karl was talking about? Maybe she was successful after all? And maybe she shouldn't concentrate directly on it. She would try it again right now.

"It worked, Karl! I heard and saw him!" Susanne was exited when she ran towards Karl. She didn't wait for him to say hello, but bubbled over with the news. "I saw Sven. He was wearing normal clothes and he smiled. Then he told me that he was OK and I shouldn't worry about him. And what is more, he is always with me and not really gone at all." Susanne beamed at the old man. Her eyes sparkled with happiness. Karl just nodded as he always did. "I told you. He is here."

Susanne blinked; then she rubbed her right eye. The sunflowers appeared blurry and their colours dull. Not as vibrant as she knew them. She had been noticing this change for quite some time. She hadn't told her parents, who were preoccupied with themselves anyway. Sometimes it seemed as though everything was shrouded in fog. Another time, she would be so sensitive to light that she had to wear sunglasses even if it was overcast. This had been going on for several days now and it wouldn't get better. She was worried.

"Can you see something in my eye, Karl?" Susanne looked at him with wide-open eyes. The right eye started running immediately. Today, her eyes were very sensitive again.

Karl thoughtfully touched his chin. "Your eye looks as though it would lose its colour, somehow gray. Do you have any other problems?" Susanne told him every little detail. How she tripped up on the step at school the other day, how the sunflowers had lost their colour, or how she didn't dare to cross the street because everything was blurry and foggy.

Karl listened carefully. "Don't you want to go to the doctor?" "But then I have to tell my parents," Susanne hummed and hawed. "I don't want to bother them even more." Karl swayed his head pensively. "But it will be hard for you if your eyes get worse." "Then they'll maybe notice it, I can't help it," said Susanne and waved aside Karl's remark. She looked at him fearfully. "Do you think I will get blind?" Karl shook his head. "No, I think your eyes will improve again. But I also think it won't be easy for you."

It took several weeks before Susanne's eyes got better again. In the meantime, she had adapted to the limitations to a certain degree. At school, she pretended to have an inflammation of the eyes when it was really bad, and the teachers believed her, because sometimes her right eye did look inflamed.

When her eyesight improved again, she almost couldn't believe it. "It is much better, Karl. I can see the true colours again and barely any fog." Susanne stood in front of him, craned her head towards him, and asked him, "Can you see anything?" Karl checked her eyes long and thoroughly. Then he nodded as he always did. "I think you are over it. Your eye is looking good again."

That night, Susanne talked to Sven. After all, she knew he was there, even though she couldn't see or hear him. She told him about Karl, her eyes, their parents, and about school. Finally, she smiled into the darkness and added, "But, actually, you know all these things anyway, right? After all, you are always with me."

Conflict and Resolution

Susanne suffered a severe visual separation conflict when her brother suddenly died. She wanted to see him, but she couldn't, because he had drowned.

In this situation, people "search" the other person with their eyes, but they don't find him or her. He or she "receded too far into the distance." The biological meaning of seeing sharply serves that purpose in the conflict active phase.

During the conflict active phase, necroses develop in the lens. As soon as the conflict is resolved, a cataract occurs. In most cases, if there continues to be only one conflict, the lens will in most cases clear up again completely.

However, repeated relapses can lead to blindness. Susanne resolved her conflict when she presumably dreamed of her brother and took the dream as proof that Sven wasn't entirely lost to her. After the resolution of the conflict through the dream, the cataract occurred. Susanne's conflict remained resolved. Relapses are unlikely.

A Hairy Affair
• Saskia and the pyelitis

"How could you do that?" Saskia felt her anger grow into rage. Angrily, she looked at her mother in law, who didn't seem to feel guilty at all. Indignantly, she lifted her eyebrows. "Do you want to let the girl run around like that? That wasn't a haircut, that was a mop," she added disparagingly. "Nele, please go outside to your father." Saskia squeezed the words out. The three-year-old girl was startled, but she obeyed. When she had left the room, Saskia turned to her mother in law again. She flashed her eyes at her. "Don't ever dare to cut Nele's hair again. Ever. Otherwise, this was the last time she visited you. I have good friends who can take better care of her." With these words, she turned around and left the room.

Saskia was still seething inside. She couldn't believe what a nerve this woman had. She had agreed for her mother in law to have her daughter over the weekend. When Nele arrived at her grandma's she had had long hair, and she returned with short hair. Lutz kept silent in the car. He felt heavy-hearted. When Saskia was in a mood like this, he would better leave her alone. He could perfectly understand his wife. What his mother had done was simply inexcusable. And the most intolerable was the fact that she seemed to be oblivious to her mistake. She had even been offended by Saskia's reaction.

"Mom, are you angry with grandma?" Nele looked at her mother attentively. "No, I am just sad that your hair was cut," Saskia said and ran her fingers through her daughter's short, blond hair. "But I like it, mom. It doesn't hurt any more when I brush it," Nele answered and tousled her hair. Then she started laughing and tousled her mother's hair as well. They romped around for a while before Saskia put Nele to bed, tucked her in, and gave her a kiss. "Not for long, princess. Soon, your hair will have grown again. Sweet dreams."

"You have to talk to her. I won't go through something like this again," Saskia demanded. Lutz sighed. "I know, sweetheart, sometimes she is impossible. But she doesn't take me seriously." Saskia looked at him. "She will take me seriously. I've had enough of her constantly interfering with our life."

"No, Nele won't visit you either tomorrow or the day after tomorrow, and in the next weeks to come either. I can't take it any more. It is our life. And if you can't accept that, you have to live with the consequences." Saskia was almost surprised about herself, how well she managed to talk to her mother in law in this manner. But she had sworn to herself to speak out this time and she would see it through.

"What is the matter, sweetheart?" Lutz looked at his wife with concern. Her face contorted with pain, she had leaned against the wall. Her hand touched the left side of her back. "Kidney pain," she said. "Is it bad?" Lutz hugged her. "I'm OK," responded Saskia. "I am going to bed." With her hand at her back she went towards the bedroom.

"Pyelitis is not to be taken lightly," the doctor said and put his instruments back into his bag. Saskia didn't even bother to nod. Lutz stood at her bedside and was worried. "I hope you have someone who can take care of your little girl. I don't think you can manage on your own while your husband is at

124

work," the doctor continued. Lutz nodded. Saskia shot a warning look at him. "Of course," she said. "What are friends for?"

"Ulla will take care of Nele," Saskia said, "at least for one or two days until I feel better." She pointed to her notebook. "Her number is in there." Wearily, she sank back into her pillow. She had taken a painkiller, and the doctor had given her antibiotics. Now she was desperate for some sleep.

Lutz let the phone ring for a while, but nobody answered. He was unnerved as he hung up. What should he do now? Ulla wasn't at home, it was already evening, and he had to find someone for Nele. He thought for a moment before he dialed his mother's number. "Mom, can you take care of Nele again? Saskia has pyelitis and I can't find anyone for her. And tomorrow morning, I have to go on a business trip that I can't cancel. Would you please do that for me?" Lutz took a deep breath. There was no going back now.

"Well, you changed your mind quickly, that's for sure," he heard his mother say at the other end. "But now that you need somebody, I am good enough again all of a sudden," she added snappishly. "But woe betide me if I do something madam doesn't like. Then I hear right away, that's it...." Unnervedly, Lutz held the receiver away from his ear. He just let her talk. At some point, she would be finished. He just didn't know yet how to explain the whole thing to Saskia. And right now, he didn't even want to think about it.

Eventually, his mother had taken Nele. That was clear from the start. Lutz didn't tell Saskia about it. She had still been a little sleepy when he said goodbye. He answered her question about Nele briefly. "She is been taken care of. And now you have to get better," he said. Then he took his daughter and was on his way.

Saskia felt much better already. She must have more or less slept through two days. The pain was mostly gone. Now she had to find out how Nele was doing. She picked up the phone, dialed Ulla's number, and waited. Nobody answered. After trying three times, she gave up. Maybe they had gone for a walk. Only when she still hadn't reached anyone at 8:00 p.m. did she start to worry. It was impossible for them to still be outside. Lutz hadn't called yet either. She felt downright abandoned.

Without further ado, she dialed Lutz's cell phone number. She was lucky. After three rings, he picked up. He seemed to be glad to hear her voice. "How are you doing, sweetheart?" "Actually, I feel OK, but I can't reach Ulla. She wouldn't be still outside with Nele at this time. Did she say anything?"

"Oh..., that." Lutz paused and took a deep breath. "Nele isn't at Ulla's, she is at my mother's. And before you say anything, I didn't have a choice; Ulla didn't answer her phone and I had to find someone quick. So, I asked my mother. I thought that was the best solution." Saskia was silent. Lutz could hear her breathe. "Sweetheart? You do understand, don't you? I mean, what was I supposed to do?" "It's OK," Saskia said. "You are right, you didn't have a choice. I see you tomorrow." With these words she hung up slowly.

"Mom, mom, look what grandma gave me!" Beaming with joy, Nele ran towards her mother. Behind her, Lutz walked self-consciously into the door, carrying a scooter. It was one of these colourful scooters with a small saddle, which was actually a little too big for Nele. Lutz shrugged his shoulders, he and Saskia looked at each other. "It is beautiful," Saskia said slowly. Then, Nele had a lot she wanted to tell her mother.

"What is she thinking?" Saskia was angry again. It wasn't Lutz's fault, but they had to find a solution. The scooter had the right size for a five-year-old, but it was much too big for Nele. What was more, her mother in law had taken a big joy away from them.

Nele was supposed to get a small scooter for her fourth birthday. They had already bought one; it was hidden in the attic. Even if they would still give it to her, Nele wouldn't be as thrilled about it. After all, she already had a big scooter, even though she couldn't ride it.

"What is she thinking, giving Nele all these gifts? How is Nele supposed to learn that she can't have everything she wants? How can we raise her when your mother is constantly interfering? I just don't know what to do." Saskia looked at Lutz helplessly. He hugged her and promised, "We will think of something."

"Two weeks? Two weeks on Hiddensee Island, just like that? Will you even get time off?" Saskia was overwhelmed. Slowly, a smile appeared on her face. Then she flung her arms around his neck. "Only the three of us on the little island. You are a genius."

"I suspect a relapse. Did you take all your medication as you were supposed to?" Reproachfully, the doctor looked at Saskia. She nodded, "I took everything as you had prescribed and as it was written on the box. I emptied the box completely." "Well, anyway, you suffer from pyelitis again. But this time, it has to heal up," the doctor demanded. Saskia nodded. She would do her best.

"I'll be fine," Saskia said to Lutz and nodded encouragingly. "Nele will stay here, it is not that bad this time. And don't even think of taking her to your mother again." Lutz smiled. "I would never do that." Then he kissed her." "Now get better quickly. After all, we want to go to the island," he reminded her. "Aye, aye, sir," she answered and raised her hand as if she was saluting. "Ouch." She winced. She quickly put her hand on her back again and looked at Lutz self-consciously. "I will manage. After all, I still have six days to recover before we leave."

126

Conflict and Resolution

Saskia suffered a conflict of territory marking when her mother in law cut her daughter's hair single-handedly without talking to her.

The conflict content is "Someone is interfering with my affairs." It is always a particular person and always the same person for a conflict as well.

During the conflict active phase, necroses, that is, cell decrease, develop in the mucosa of the renal pelvis. If any, they cause mild dragging pain in the kidney area.

In the healing phase, pyelitis is diagnosed while the necroses are being filled. Many patients have kidney stones as well. The renal colic represents the epileptoid crisis.

Saskia resolved her conflict after she had made it clear to her mother in law, that she wouldn't accept her interfering any longer. When Lutz had to take Nele to his mother again, and she interfered again with how they raised their daughter, Saskia suffered a relapse. She will only be able to ultimately resolve the conflict if she finds a way to prevent her mother in law from interfering in the future.

Late Freedom
• Anne and the stroke

She looked around in her comfortable one-bedroom apartment with pride. It looked good, she decided. Anne had bought new furniture for the entire apartment after she had left Klaus just three months ago. Finally, she had done it. She still couldn't believe it. After 30 years of marriage and three children, she had left her husband. "And I should have done it much earlier," she thought. "I would have spared us a lot." She picked up a book, sat down in a chair on her new balcony, and started to read.

Not only had Anne moved out, but she had also chosen a different location. Her new home was a little village 15 kilometers from the city. Now, she took the bus to work and back every day. And although that was strenuous, she felt good. At first, her unfamiliar freedom felt strange. She didn't have to consider anyone else's needs any more, neither her children's nor Klaus's. She could do whatever she wanted whenever she wanted to do it. She got along very well with her new neighbours. And she didn't even mind any more when Klaus visited her every day at work. After he had learned very quickly that she wouldn't change her mind, he didn't try to convince her any further. "Actually, we get along better now than ever before. This way, our marriage could have worked," Anne thought.

"Your apartment is very comfortable and really nice." Christian nodded appreciatively before he hugged his mother. "And how are you feeling?" Attentively, he looked her in the eyes. She beamed at him. "You know, son, it is wonderful. Of course, I have a long way to get to work, but everything else is perfect. And you know what is the best of all? Finally, I have dreams again."

"Dreams? What do you mean?" asked Christian. "Just normal dreams, during my sleep. I haven't dreamed in a very long time. I used to have so many colourful dreams. I need dreaming to feel relaxed."

Christian remembered those times very well. Sometimes, she had actually told him about her dreams. For example, the one where she had dreamed to be a witch in the middle ages who was burned. He laughed. "Considering your dreams, I would be glad not to have any. Think of the witch burning." Anne laughed as well. "Well, except for such nightmares, of course." Then she became serious. "I acted too late, much too late." Unsure how he should react, Christian averted his eyes. Then he looked at her again. "Better late than never. You'll see, from now on things can only get better."

His mother's voice on the phone sounded depressed. Christian realized it, however, he didn't ask a respective question. He simply hadn't the time right now. His sons were still up although it was already 10:00 p.m. and he still had to work on his project. "It's OK, son," Anne said. "I am just keeping you. Say hello to the boys for me. I am looking forward to see you in October."

Later, when he was lying in bed, Christian thought about the call again. He pondered, "Is it possible that she is sad because she is alone? Maybe she underestimated the extent of the whole situation." After all, she had never lived alone. From her parents she had gone straight into a marriage she actually didn't really want. But after the second illegitimate child she wouldn't

128

postpone it any longer. The social pressure had been too much. So, she had married Klaus, his father. "That was a big mistake," Christian thought once again. "They don't have anything in common."

His father was a quiet man, a loner. He was unhappy in his job as a police officer and, oftentimes, he took his anger out on Anne. Anne, on the other hand, was fun loving and extrovert. She made friends quickly and reacted sensitive when someone answered back. Then she would start yelling. She had been quick in slapping Christian and his brothers. His father had kept out of it. He had complained about his sons with his mother when he didn't like something.

Later, he drank alcohol more and more frequently and had become cantankerous. For nights on end Christian had heard them fighting. Often, they would insult each other deeply when they thought the children were asleep. Christian had wished they would separate, but they had never done it. "I can't raise you without his money. I don't earn enough," she once admitted to Christian after he had asked her.

Christian's thoughts wandered again. Today, she had been depressed. Like sometimes in the past. And he had not have time for her. Suddenly he blamed himself. "I'll give her a call tomorrow, absolutely." And with this thought on his mind, he fell asleep.

Christian didn't forget. Relieved, he listened to his mother, who had told him now uninterruptedly for the last five minutes about her neighbour and also about the new colleague she was training. Although the names didn't mean anything to him, he was assuaged by her energy. After half an hour, he passed the receiver on to Finn, his eldest son. He was his grandmother's favourite. He was twelve years old and a rather introverted boy. Carl was the complete opposite. When Finn called with his grandmother on the phone, he came out of his shell. He loved her very much.

Christian had just walked into the door when the phone rang. He picked up. It was his father, who spoke in a choked voice, and before Christian could think about it, he learned the reason. "Come home, son, your mom suffered a stroke today, a severe stroke. She is in a coma and doesn't react at all. I don't know how long she will make it." Christian was numb. "A stroke?" Then his eyes filled with tears. "No problem. I'll be there as soon as possible."

Christian had planned to visit his mother during the fall break anyway. The boys had been looking forward to it for weeks; they wanted to leave tomorrow. Now they would arrive a day earlier than they had planned. But what was awaiting them? Christian had a hard time holding back his tears. His mother wasn't even 60 years old.

Finn and Carl sat quietly in the car. When Christian looked in the rearview mirror, he saw tears running down the cheeks of his twelve-year-old son. Obviously, just like Christian, he was worried that his grandma could die before they arrived.

Five hours later, they arrived in the little village. Christian dropped the boys off at his father's before he drove to the hospital. Christian had been raising the boys by himself since they were in kindergarten. When they were divorced, his wife didn't show any interest in them. "Hello, brother." Steffen, his younger brother stood in front of him. His eyes lay deep in their sockets, he seemed lost. They hugged each other without a word. "How is she doing?" Christian asked quietly. "Not good," Steffen answered. "She is still in a coma."

Christian decided not to let his sons see their grandmother. Not as long as she was on all these drips, in a hemiplegic state, and not responsive. He had had the same experience with his grandmother. He had been horrified and he would have preferred to remember her in a different way. Finn and Carl accepted his decision. Neither of them questioned it. They stayed with their grandfather when Christian and Steffen were visiting their mother. Their eldest brother had been visiting only for a day before he drove home again.

Day after day, both men were sitting at her mother's bed. They read to her from a book that Christian knew she would like. But he wasn't sure whether she understood anything. She still wouldn't react, but sometimes it appeared as though her heartbeat would slow down while they were reading to her. Christian was still hoping, although the doctor only shook his head. "Your mother doesn't have very much of a chance. The brain pressure increased, but we can't do surgery. Even if she survived, the damage would be massive."

When the phone rang this time, Christian knew it was the hospital. "It has been 13 days," he thought. "She has been in a coma for 13 days," he repeated in his thoughts. "Hello," he answered the phone in a low voice. "Your mother passed away this morning shortly after 7:00 a.m.," said the doctor at the other end. Christian hung up slowly.

Conflict and Resolution

"Better late than never" Christian says to his mother, but he is only conditionally right. In fact, some conflicts are not to be resolved in order not to risk a person's death.

That applies primarily if the conflict has been going on for a very long time. In Anne's case, it has probably lasted for 30 years. She was trapped in a marriage with a man she couldn't leave, because she didn't want to risk the well being of her children.

Although she and Klaus didn't love each other, fought a lot, and were unhappy with one another, they stayed together. Only when her children had moved out and Anne couldn't bear it any longer did she separate from her husband, moved, and started a new life. In the process, she resolved her motor conflict.

If the Hamer Focus, which can range into the motor cortex, is very big as a result of the healing, it becomes dangerous. It puts pressure on the brain, ultimately leading to palsy.

The stroke is the epileptoid crisis. We don't know the exact DHS, that is, the second the conflict started. Anne must have experienced a so-called motor conflict, a situation, in which she couldn't escape her husband. After that, the conflict possibly went on this track for 30 years.

A Strong Moment
• Mark and the glaucoma

Again, he felt the ruler in his back. He leaned forward anxiously. The teacher could not notice anything, because if he did, Mark was called to the blackboard immediately. He already knew that. Mr. Merkel didn't like him. So far, Mark hadn't been able to find out why the teacher couldn't stand him. That's just how it was. He couldn't change anything about it.

He could hear the malicious hissing behind him. "Little Mark, come, little Mark, let us brush your hair. It is so golden and so soft." Now he could already hear louder snorting behind him. Ralf and Konrad had a whale of a time at his expense.

As he was trying to lean forward even further to avoid the ruler, Mark accidentally knocked his pencil case off the table. Mr. Merkel reacted to the noise instantly. "Ah, I realize we have a volunteer. Well, why don't you come to the blackboard and explain the equation to us." Obviously, that was too much for his tormentors. They almost fell off their chairs with laughter. "Yes, Mark," Konrad added, "Explain the world to us, sweetie." Now the entire class was laughing. Except for Lissy. She drew something in her notebook. The teacher pretended not to hear anything. He looked towards Mark. Then he nodded towards the blackboard.

Mark was hiding in his secret corner. The two idiots wouldn't find him here. His hiding place was directly beside the schoolyard. Mark squeezed through a hole in the fence to reach it. On the other side was an overgrown garden, no one was living there and nobody saw him. He had his peace here. However, he had to be careful not to get caught. It was forbidden to leave the schoolyard. If they caught him, he would get a bad mark, which he really didn't need. He needed good grades to be able to go to high school. These two idiots wouldn't be able to follow him there. That was his only rescue.

Mark couldn't sleep. He stared into the darkness and pondered. He had to do something. It just couldn't go on like this. Ralf and Konrad were constantly bullying him. Not only during lessons and recess, but recently, they were also waiting for him after school. They had even trapped him in front of his house. Apparently, they had a lot of fun following him. Mark didn't feel safe anywhere except for his room and his secret hiding place. Everywhere else, he felt pursued. He couldn't tell his parents about it. His father would just contemptuously wrinkle his nose and boast about his fights. His mother would run to the teachers and complain, which would make things even worse. Mark had to think of something.

Mark rubbed his arm. Konrad was pretty strong. Again and again, he hit him on his upper arm whenever he felt like it, often even during lessons. He always hit the same spot. Mark couldn't remember the last time he didn't have a bruise on his arm. Today, it was particularly bad. Because Mark endured the blows with stoic indifference, Ralf changed his tactics. He stepped in front of him and hit him in the stomach without any warning. Then he watched Mark squirm. When Mark was able to stand up straight again to a certain degree, he hit him again. Mark could barely breathe.

Half-heartedly, he tried to hit back. But Konrad held his hand down and hissed maliciously, "You will pay for this, little Mark. You raised your hand against us? That will be costly. You better bring five Euros if you don't want the same treatment again tomorrow." His mouth was very close to Mark's face; Mark could smell onions and turned his head in disgust. Angrily, Konrad turned Mark's head back again. "Hey, you stay where you are, Shorty. Did you get me?" While he was talking, Konrad's saliva sprayed all over Mark's face. He couldn't turn his head away. He nodded quickly. Then, Konrad pushed him away. "Don't forget it, Mark." Mark looked crestfallen when he walked away. From the corner of his eyes he saw Lissy watching him. She stood there quietly and looked at him.

Absent-mindedly, Mark sat at his desk and stared out of the window. Sometimes, his eyes fell on Lissy. He was a little in love with her, but he would never let on. Subconsciously, he was constantly awaiting new attacks from the desk behind him. But his tormentors were busy. His class was writing a test, and this time they couldn't even copy from him. He had already handed his sheet to Mr. Merkel, who had collected it without commenting. Mark was thinking. As always, it was about the one topic: How could he get rid of these two guys? It would be another four months until the new school year started and they went their separate ways, but he had to find a solution before that, or he would go crazy.

"Where is the money, little Mark?" Mark froze. He hadn't expected to run into them so quickly. He had just entered the schoolyard. That didn't leave him any chance to escape.

"Uhm, guys, about the money…." Angrily, the two boys walked towards him. "What?" asked Konrad and looked at him in disgust. "You probably need the money for your facial care, right? So that you can treat your pimples." He pointed maliciously at Mark's face where big pimples were sprouting since the other day. Automatically, Mark touched them. Then he concentrated again on his plan.

He thought about it briefly, but then he bubbled over, "I couldn't get the money, but I have cigarettes, three boxes. You can have those." Now he paused. Konrad and Ralf looked at each other; then they grinned. "Give them to us." "OK, come with me. I hid them." Mark walked quickly in front of them. He looked for the supervising teacher. He spotted the gym teacher. That was good; he was impartial and fair. It could work.

Mark led the two boys to his hiding place. If his plan went wrong, his hideout would burn down. But he had to take that risk. He was about to squeeze through the hole when Ralf grabbed him. "You wait here. First, I go, then you, and then Konni." He wriggled through the hole. Mark and Konrad followed him. Mark had another quick look at the schoolyard. The gym teacher, Mr. Timm, was only about ten meters away.

Determinedly, he led both of them to the garden, directly to a dilapidated wall. "Under here," Mark said and began to clear a few bricks. "Stop, goldilocks," Konrad said. "We'll do it. How knows what else you have there." Mark nodded, seemingly scared; however, inside he was grinning. "They fall for my line completely." Ralf and Konrad cleared a few more bricks. Mark used that opportunity, started running like a bolt of lightning, disappeared through the fence, saw the gym teacher and shouted, "Mr. Timm, Mr. Timm, I think two students are in trouble over there!" The gym teacher reacted instinctively and ran to the hole Mark showed him. Before he could say anything, Konrad and Ralf appeared in the hole.

Angrily, they flashed their eyes at Mark. "Everything is OK. We are fine," they assured the gym teacher, who looked suspiciously at them and then at the wall and decided, "You come with me, both of you." He didn't pay any attention to Mark. Walking past Mark, Konrad hissed, "We'll get you, little Mark." Mark knew what would follow. The two of them had to explain why they had been in the forbidden area and they would be punished. The important thing was that the gym teacher played his part. Mark waited nervously. Only two more minutes before recess was over.

There he was. Mr. Timm walked right up to Mark who pretended not to notice him. "Why did you call for help, Mark?" Mr. Timm looked at him sternly. Mark shrugged his shoulders. "It seemed strange. I was worried. There appeared to be smoke and I heard rocks cracking. Then I saw someone. It was a reflex," he said with an innocent expression on his face. The teacher observed him attentively. Then he squeezed through the hole in the fence and walked to the wall to examine it. He lifted several bricks, looked underneath, and inspected the hole in the wall. Mark crossed his fingers. Suddenly, the gym teacher came back. He held a small bag in his hand. Mark was jumping for joy inside. The teacher had found it, his plan had worked out.

Ralf and Konrad were kicked out of school; they each had to go to another school. "Grade eight students with cannabis, that is absolutely outrageous," the principal commented at a school meeting in front of everybody. "The more so as the two boys obviously planned on dealing drugs; they used that garden as their warehouse, so it seems." He had wiped his sweaty forehead. "I don't know what to say. I can only hope the press won't find out. Thirteen-year-old boys dealing with hashish!" Mark almost had to grin. Was this man living under a rock? Drugs had almost become normal in the meantime and hardly anybody made a big deal out of it. Too bad, though, if you got caught.

Mark actually did have a part in Ralf and Konrad getting caught. He had watched them the afternoon before the action, followed them, and, that way, found the place where they were hiding the drugs. A few of the little bags were enough to blow the whistle on them. Secretly, he was expecting for them to take bloody revenge. But when he met them two days later, they looked at him almost scared. As if they didn't know what to think of him. Mark didn't care. He didn't even care about being beaten up by them one more time. Soon, they would be too busy with working their community service hours anyway.

Mechanically, he touched his cheek. The pimples were gone, and he didn't even have to treat them. "Not bad," he thought. But recently, he was suffering from a pretty bad headache. He blinked and tried to read what Mr. Merkel had written on the blackboard. Now, even his eyes were hurting. The teacher noticed that something was going on with Mark. He watched him attentively. "I can see how interested you are and I don't want to be in the way. I hereby invite you to come to the blackboard."

Mark barely managed to get home. There, he ran to the bathroom and threw up. The headache had gotten bad towards the end of the school day and so did the eye pain. Now he felt better, although he still felt a little nauseated.

Mark lay down. Some sleep would probably help. Mark was right, at least partly. When his mother noticed two hours later that he was voluntarily taking a nap, she became suspicious. "I'm OK, really," Mark tried to convince her, but it was in vain. His mother called the doctor, who came by a little while later. After a short examination, he gave him a sick note. "Probably a virus infection," he said. "I can't tell for sure, but the symptoms point to it. You better stay in bed for a few days." Then he thought about it briefly and added, "For a week, I would say."

"You have a visitor, Mark," he heard his mother's voice through the door. Mark quickly put the book away. The door opened. Mark was surprised to see Lissy. "Hey, what are you doing here?" he asked in astonishment. "I brought your homework," Lissy answered.

She walked over to the table, took a few notebooks out of her bag and put them on his desk cover. Mark still looked completely surprised. "When will you come back to school?" Lissy sat down on the edge of the bed and looked at him attentively with her green eyes. Mark felt how he blushed. "Tomorrow, I think. Yes, tomorrow for sure." Lissy grinned. "Quite an eager beaver, aren't you? Tomorrow is Sunday."

Conflict and Resolution

Mark suffered a fear-breathing-down-his-neck conflict; in his case, it was the fear of a person rather than a thing. Ralf and Konrad were constantly after Mark, and he felt as though he had Konrad, who was the leader, on his back all the time. Konrad was lying in wait for Mark everywhere Mark went.

During the conflict active phase, the vitreous body of the eye becomes blurred. Once the conflict is resolved, the opacity of the vitreous body degenerates with the development of a vitreous edema, which is the so-called glaucoma. Glaucoma means a pressure increase inside the eye. The conflict becomes dangerous if there are repeated relapses. In that case, the internal eye pressure remains high and damages the optic nerve, which can lead to blindness.

Mark resolved his conflict quickly and subsequently suffered an acute glaucoma attack, which remained undetected as such. Instead, the doctor assumed a virus infection.

Furthermore, Mark suffered a defilement conflict when Konrad's saliva sprayed over his face. He developed pimples, which serve to particularly protect, that is, strengthen the skin in those areas that came in contact with the saliva. The pimples cleared up once Mark's tormentors had left the school. There are other kinds of pimples as well, which can also develop from the connective tissue as a result of a collapse of self-esteem.

Incidentally, glaucoma is frequently detected during preventive medical checkups in people 40 years and older.

If Mark had suffered a conflict of fear breathing down his neck of a thing, he would probably have become shortsighted. In such cases, cell decomposition occurs in the photoreceptors of the retina area during the conflict active phase, and in the healing phase the retina peels away from the eye. The healing edema visually lengthens the eyeball because the ability to focus decreases as a result of the scarring. The person becomes shortsighted.

Regarding the Case Studies

- Acknowledgements
- Instructions

We would like to thank all those affected who were willing to reveal their very personal stories. We especially thank the practitioners of the New Medicine who helped us choose the cases and present the diagnosis.

Now it is up to you to decide what you as the reader will do with the information. Using the case studies as examples, the authors would like to provide you with a broader basis to form your own opinion. If you agree with or reject Hamer's New Medicine based on emotional reasons, you should distrust your judgment. Science doesn't have an emotional aspect. If it isn't rational, it isn't science; it's either religion or opinion.

That's why we haven't included Dr. Ryke Geerd Hamer's personal story or the relatively new name for his discovery, *Germanic New Medicine®*, which is protected by the trademark law. For, science knows neither sympathy nor antipathy. It is never right or wrong based on emotions, but provable or disprovable based on facts. Scientists can be persecuted; science can be disproved at best. Science knows neither race nor religion or nationality. It is either generally accepted or it isn't science, as the expert opinion regarding the New Medicine by Prof. Dr. Hans-Ulrich Niemitz stresses in the first factor-L book.

And please do not forget: Try to avoid the "isolation" factor. Visit forums, stay or get in contact with others. Always exchange your opinion with other people. If you ignore other opinions, you deprive yourself of the chance to check your own.

Reading tip:
faktor-L. Neue Medizin.
Die Wahrheit über Dr. Hamers Entdeckung
Krebs und andere heilbare Krankheiten
Monika Berger-Lenz * Christopher Ray * Prof. Dr. H. U. Niemitz
ISBN: 3-9809203-9-9
EAN: 9783980920391

***

English Translation
In Preparation for Publication:
factor-L* New Medicine
The Truth about Dr. Hamer's Discovery
Cancer and other curable diseases
Monika Berger-Lenz * Christopher Ray * Prof. Dr. H. U. Niemitz

Glossary
of the
New Medicine

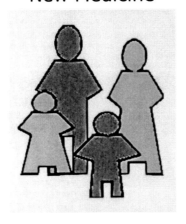

A Reference guide for the New Medicine
according to Dr. Ryke Geerd Hamer

***

A Special Thank you for their support
to Patricia, Regine, and Antje

***

Note in regard to extent and validity:
Knowledge has no final aspect!
This glossary presents a snapshot
of the currently available knowledge in regard to the New Medicine
and is not exhaustive, or permanently accurate.

Acromegaly
Growth of the nose, toes, chin, ears, etc. in adults due to a pituitary tumor. See there.

Acute hearing loss
Temporary deafness regarding the affected sound frequencies during the PCL phase; infusions are counterproductive, because edemas are developed during the hearing phase.
See also: Tinnitus

Addison's disease
See: Cushing's syndrome

Adenocarcinoma
Cauliflower-like tumors

Adenoids
Nasopharyngeal adenoids

DHS conflict content:
Left side: "being unable to get rid of a chunk"
Right side: "being unable to grasp a chunk"

CA phase: Developments of adenoids

PCL phase: In most cases smelly caseating of the adenoids through fungi and mycobacteria

Adiposity
(Obesity, overweight)
See:
Diabetes
Syndrome

Adrenal cortex insufficiency
See: Cushing's syndrome

Adult Onset Diabetes
See: Diabetes

Allergy
A SBS that occurs not because of a DHS but due to a track someone is set on over and over again.
See:
SBS
Track
Conflict resolution

Alzheimer's Disease
The underlying conflicts with "Alzheimer's Disease" are always separation conflicts, mostly physical right side and left side (partner and child/mother), i.e., also in both brain hemispheres (so-called constellation), that is, in the sensory (skin) and post-sensory (periosteum) cortex center. Long lasting or frequently relapsing separation conflicts virtually lead to brain cirrhosis, i.e., the brain somewhat contracts, particularly at the location of the conflict relay. Thus, it seems as if the skullcap is a little too big for the brain. But even "Alzheimer's Disease" is not a mistake of nature, but "intentional forgetting". In nature, this "need to forget" is often vital for the survival. But that won't change the fact that it is very sad having to watch such biological behaviour patterns in the extreme example.

In the traditional medicine they talk in regards to Alzheimer's about an atrophy of the cerebral cortex (tissue loss) with various symptoms. Disturbances of memory, disorientation, speech impediments, affected intellectual power, and impaired consciousness.

According to Dr. Hamer, these symptoms of Alzheimer's Disease reflect the "ravages of time". In the process, the Hamer Foci play a central role. Due to many Hamer Foci scarred over during a lifetime (that can be different conflicts), the brain shrinks, which affects the relays to the point of "dysfunctions" (uncontrolled movements).

The typical "symptoms" like the lack of the short-term memory and forgetfulness are caused by the described separation conflicts and their relapses. The characteristic here: The Hamer Foci are each in the sensory and post-sensory cortex of the same hemisphere.

Amelanotic Melanoma
See: Melanoma

Angina Pectoris
See: Heart Attack

Ankle joint pain
DHS conflict content: SWE of "not being able to walk, dance, or balance"

Example:
CA phase: Bone osteolyses in this area, anemia

PCL phase: Edema and expansion of the periosteum, pain, recalcification, leukemia, and joint rheumatism (in traditional medicine often: arthritis)

The recalcification corresponds with the diagnosis of the traditional medicine: osteosarcoma

Germ layer: Mesoderm
See also: SWE

Aphthous oral infection
Thrush

DHS conflict content: "Being unable to grasp the chunk"

Example:
When severely ill people can't ingest food properly any longer, or small children having to "beg" for the next spoonful of food

CA phase: Barely visible, flat adenocarcinoma under the mucous membrane of the squamous epithelium in the mouth

PCL phase: Aphthous oral infection, thrush fungus of the mouth

Germ layer: Endoderm, attributed to the brain stem

Appendicitis
DHS conflict content: Nasty indigestible anger

Example: A child/student is severely reprimanded and punished by the teacher because of a small, unintentional misbehaviour without being able to oppose.

CA phase: Cauliflower-like appendix carcinoma

PCL phase: Appendicitis.
Appendix rupture: During the CA phase the carcinoma blocked the appendix; therefore, it can rupture in the PCL-phase.

Germ layer - Endoderm

Arthritis
See: SWE

Asthma
Bronchial Asthma
Laryngeal Asthma

DHS conflict content: A so-called constellation exists. Mostly a hanging conflict ("downtransformed" but constantly active); constant, mostly weaker relapses, possibly also on tracks.

Handedness:
Right-handed woman:
Conflict 1 – fear due to shock (larynx), conflict 2 – another conflict of the cerebrum, for example, threat to the territory (bronchi) (experienced in a male fashion during conflict 2, as female side is blocked by conflict 1)

Left-handed woman
Conflict 1 – fear due to shock (bronchi), conflict 2 - another conflict of the cerebrum, for example, fear due to shock (larynx) (can experience the same conflict twice, as male side of the brain is blocked by conflict 1)

Right-handed man:

Conflict 1 – threat to the territory (bronchi), conflict 2 - another conflict of the cerebrum, for example, fear due to shock (larynx) (experienced in a female fashion during conflict 2, as male side is blocked by conflict 1)

Left-handed man:
Conflict 1 – threat to the territory (larynx), conflict 2 - another conflict of the cerebrum, for example, threat to the territory (bronchi) (can experience the same conflict twice, as female side of the brain was blocked by conflict 1)

Attention: In addition to the handedness, the hormonal state also influences that side of the brain, in which the impact occurs. See also: Handedness.

Example: A right-handed boy is constantly under strict control of his mother, she constantly violates his privacy; she possibly also reads his diary, his mail, enters his room unexpectedly, etc.

Conflict active (CA) phase: If both conflicts are in the CA phase: expiratory wheezing, prolonged exhaling (bronchial asthma), prolonged inhaling (laryngeal asthma)

141

Post-conflictolytic (PCL) phase: If one conflict (bronchial or larynx relay) is in the process of being resolved and the other one is in the CA phase, an asthma attack (bronchial or laryngeal) occurs in the epileptic crisis of the resolved conflict.

Epileptic crisis of both conflicts at the same time, if they are located in the bronchial- as well as the larynx relay: Acute asthmatic shortness of breath!

Germ layer: Ectoderm

Astigmatism
See: Irregular curvature of the cornea

Atrophy
Atrophy (Greek: ill-nourished, atrophy, without food) means loss of tissue. It can occur through a decrease in cell size (hypotrophy) or loss of cells (hypoplasy), each with or without simultaneous alterations in the cell structure.

Back pain

(Spinal pain)

Rheumatism

DHS conflict content: Central personality SWE

CA phase: Bone osteolyses in this area

PCL phase: Edema and expansion of the periosteum, pain, recalcification, and leukemia

Germ layer: Mesoderm
See also: SWE

Basedow's Disease
See: Thyroid dysfunctions

Benign
The most important distinguishing features between "benign" and "malignant" cells according to the traditional medicine are:

Benign cells:
- sharply differentiated
- slowly growing
- spare blood vessels
- remain encapsulated
- don't destroy surrounding tissue (not invasive = don't grow into "healthy tissue")
- don't grow again after removal

- don't develop metastases

"Benign cells" develop "benign tumors", e.g., struma, myoma, adenoma, cyst, or wart.
According the Dr. Hamer's New Medicine, the tumors categorized as "benign" rather correspond to the "repairs" controlled by the cerebral cortex (outer germ layer) of the skin, that is, the growth (cell plus) of the PCL phase AFTER the cell minus of the CA phase. Occasionally, they also correspond to the tumors controlled by the cerebellum (inner germ layer = endoderm or middle germ layer = mesoderm) in the PCL phase (healing phase). These tumors can be found in particular if there are no respective microorganisms in the body that can catabolize them.

Such an encapsulated tumor is sometimes categorized as "malignant" if another tumor was detected before. In the traditional medicine they talk in this context about "metastases".

See also:
Malignant
Metastasis
Cancer

Binge eating / self-induced vomiting
See: Bulimia nervosa

Blood pressure, high
The systolic (higher) value is too high: Active fluid conflict
(Kidney parenchyma is affected)

The diastolic (lower) value is too high: Female: conflict of "not being copulated with"
Male: territory conflict

Depending on handedness:
Concerning left-handed women or (right-handed women in constellations) it is very important to know how long the conflict lasted.

Before the conflict resolution is realized, it is absolutely necessary to involve a therapist, because the patient could suffer a heart attack (epileptic crisis) if the conflict has been active for too long.

142

Bone cancer
DHS conflict content: SWE, see under the different classifications, e.g., knee joint, back, etc.

Example:
CA phase: Bone osteolyses in this area, anemia

PCL phase: Edema and expansion of the periosteum, pain, recalcification, leukemia, and joint rheumatism (in traditional medicine often: arthritis)

The recalcification corresponds with the diagnosis of the traditional medicine: osteosarcoma

Germ layer: Mesoderm
See also: SWE

Brain tumor
What is referred to as "brain tumor", is the accumulation of connective tissue (glia) during the healing phase after the conflict resolution.

See: HH (Hamer Foci)
See also differentiation toward:
Pituitary gland tumor

Breast cancer
Mammary gland cancer
Ductal mamma carcinoma

DHS-conflict content: Mother/child conflict, daughter/mother conflict, nest conflict, worry- or argument conflict with the partner (not sexual)

Handedness:
Left breast affected:
Right-handed woman: Mother/child conflict, daughter/mother conflict, nest conflict
Left-handed woman: Worry- or argument conflict with the partner (not sexual)

Right breast affected:
Right-handed woman: Worry- or argument conflict with the partner (not sexual)
Left-handed woman: Mother/child conflict, daughter/mother conflict, nest conflict

Example: A child has an accident and the mother blames herself (mother/child conflict), or the lease of an apartment ends (nest conflict)

CA phase: Compact lump, tumor

PCL phase: Caseating decomposition with mycobacteria, or encapsulation. Pain occurs only in the last phase of the healing process.

Germ layer – Mesoderm

Characteristic: In open tumors (for example, opened through puncture), caseating, smelling decomposition, mostly accompanied by abscess development or inflammation of the breast.

See also differentiation:
Mamma carcinoma

Breathing difficulties
See:
Head cold
Bronchitis
Cough
Asthma
Pneumonia
Adenoids
Cystic Fibrosis
Bronchial Cancer
Lung Cancer

Bronchial cancer
In the epileptic crisis of bronchial cancer:
Pneumonia
See:
Bronchitis
Asthma
Pneumonia

As well as differentiation toward:
Bronchial cancer of the goblet sells in the bronchi
Cystic fibrosis
Pneumonia

Bronchial cancer of the goblet cells
In the bronchi
DHS-conflict content: Fear of suffocating, conflict of "not being able to suck in the chunk of air"

CA phase: Growth of the goblet cells in the bronchi, therefore increased secretion of fluids in order to have the "chunk of air" slide easier

PCL phase: Caseation of the adenocarcinomas of the goblet cells

Germ layer: Endoderm

Characteristic: Several relapses or occurrence in infancy can cause the complete decomposition of the goblet cells. This is how cystic fibrosis originates.

Bronchitis
Conflict content: threat to the territory and fear due to shock, depending on handedness and sex. See description under Asthma

See: Asthma

Bulbus duodeni
See: Stomach ulcer

Bulimia nervosa:
Binge eating / Self-induced vomiting

DHS conflict content: Fear-disgust conflict, territory trouble conflict, identity conflict; pay attention to constellations!

Handedness
Right-handed woman:

Conflict 1: fear-disgust conflict (hypoglycemia), conflict 2: (Because the female side of the brain is already blocked, now experienced in a male fashion, here:) - territory trouble (stomach ulcer or bile duct ulcer)

Left-handed woman:

Conflict 1: identity conflict (stomach ulcer or bile duct ulcer), conflict 2 - (Because the male side of the brain is already blocked, experienced in a female fashion again, here:) - fear-disgust conflict (hypoglycemia)

Right-handed man:

Conflict 1: territory trouble conflict (stomach ulcer or bile duct ulcer), conflict 2: (Because the male side of the brain is blocked, now experienced in a female fashion, here:) fear-disgust conflict (hypoglycemia)

Left-handed man:

Conflict 1: conflict of being reluctant (hypoglycemia), conflict 2: (Because the female side of the brain is blocked, experienced in a male fashion again, here:) territory trouble (stomach ulcer or bile duct ulcer)

Cachexia
Physical wasting

If no conflict resolution happens and the patient remains for a long time in the state of conflict (no downtransforming of the conflict mass), that is, constant sympathicotonia in the CA phase, he or she can die of exhaustion and physical wasting (cachexia in so-called cancer patients).

Calotte pain
See: Skullcap pain

Cancer
Carcinoma

It is important to know that the New Medicine won't distinguish between benign and malignant tumors. The term cancer is referring here to the events at the organ level in general. Diseases that aren't cancer in the traditional sense are considered "cancer equivalent". Hence, in the New Medicine all so-called diseases are referred to as "cancer".

The same is the case with the term "carcinoma". It doesn't use the term to describe the "malignant growth" as is done in the traditional medicine.
See also:
Benign
Malignant
Metastasis

Cancer of the tongue
Lingual- or glossal carcinoma
DHS conflict content: Speechlessness

Example:
A patient was left speechless when his boss snapped at him: "Don't you have a tongue in your mouth? Is that why you don't say a single word?"

CA phase: Abscesses, ulcers

During the CA phase, the functionally defective cells are being rejected, because they are not up for the mechanical strain. That explains the "lack of substance", the substance defect. The longer the conflict last, the bigger and deeper is the ulcer.

PCL phase: Severe local swelling, filling of the ulcers through viruses

Germ layer: (Outer) ectoderm

Hamer Focus (HH): Medio frontal basal (right or left)

CA phase
CA phase = conflict active phase

The CA phase begins directly with the DHS. It is characterized by "constant stress", cold hand and feet, and lack of appetite; the thoughts circle constantly around the conflict (sympathicotonia).

Tumors grow, necroses progress depending on the kind of conflict.

Once the conflict is resolved the CA phase ends and the PCL phase (healing phase) begins.

See also:
PCL phase
Epileptic crisis
SBS
DHS

Carcinogenic
Term from the traditional medicine
Meaning: Cancer-causing

Note: Officially, the terms carcinogen and mutagen are not used synonymously. They are, however, subject to occasional fluctuations in their use. For example, a chemical classified as "mutagen" by one producer can be categorized as "carcinogenic", or just as "poisonous" by another. Example: ethediumbromid. See the package inserts of different producers.

Carcinoma
See: Cancer

Cervical
Cervical vertebra
Regarding cancer: Cervix cancer

Chemotherapy (with cancer)
Term from the traditional medicine (SM)

"Chemotherapy" means the application of so-called "cytostatics" as treatment for so-called cancerous diseases. This group of agents prevents cell division. Hence, the cells can't multiply any more. The goal is to prevent the so-called cancer cells from multiplying.

However, chemotherapy prevents all other body cells from dividing as well, because the application can't be limited to the tumor tissue, which especially effects fast-growing tissue like mucous membranes and hair.

The application of the chemotherapy creates the image of the "typical cancer patient". The growth-repressive effect of such cytostatics is very controversial with reference to the growth of cancer tumors.

From the point of view of the "NM after Dr. Hamer": According to the NM (New Medicine), the ineffectiveness/effectiveness of the cytostasis can be traced back to the fact that chemotherapeutics are basically sympathicotonic (vegetative tonus up) and organs controlled by the cerebrum do cell multiplication including swelling only in the vagotony (parasympathicotonia). As a logical consequence, the cellular growth in organs that are controlled by the cerebrum stops with the application of chemotherapeutics.

In organs controlled by the inner germ layer (endoderm) cell multiplication occurs during the sympathycotonia, thus, chemotherapy rather causes an increase of cell growth, which goes unnoticed, of course, because a fast growing of the cells is assumed anyway.

According to Dr. Hamer, a good portion of the diagnosed cancers is an occurrence of the cerebrum, as many symptoms develop here (tonus). However, as soon as metastases are diagnosed, that is, according to the NM, "consequential conflicts", which are very often an occurrence of the inner germ layer, because they are the most archaic conflicts (fear of death or starvation, etc.), chances increasingly worsen, because these cancers grow even faster when treated with chemotherapy.

Cervical cancer
DHS conflict content: Conflict of "not being copulated with", conflict of sexual frustration

Example:
A woman catches her husband and his lover in the act.

Handedness:
Right-handed woman:
Conflict 1 – conflict of "not being copulated with" (cervical carcinoma and

simultaneously coronary vein ulcer),
epileptic crisis: pulmonary embolism -
right ventricular infarction

CA phase: Cervical tumor, amenorrhea
(no menstrual period), coronary vein
ulcer, and mild angina pectoris

PCL phase: Pulmonary embolism / right
ventricular infarction, decomposition of
cervical tumor

Handedness:
Left-handed woman:
Conflict 1 – sexual conflict (coronary
vein ulcer–carcinoma), epileptic crisis
after conflict 1: left ventricular infarction

Conflict 2 would be female side of the
brain, because the male side is blocked,
e.g., another sexual conflict (cervical
carcinoma and coronary vein ulcer–
carcinoma). Epileptic crisis after conflict
2: Right ventricular infarction
(pulmonary embolism)

CA phase: After conflict 1: Coronary
vein ulcer–carcinoma together with
depression; after conflict 2, if a sexual
conflict: Uterine tumor, coronary vein
ulcer, angina pectoris

PCL phase: After conflict 1: Left
ventricular infarction; after conflict 2:
Decomposition of the tumor, right
ventricular infarction (pulmonary
embolism)

See also:
Uterine cancer
Heart attack
Uterine catarrh
See: endometriosis
Uterine cancer
Uterine cancer

See:
Endometrial cancer
Fallopian tube cancer
Myoma
Cervical cancer
Ovarian cancer
Heart attack

Cervical canal

See also: Cervical cancer

Chicken pox

DHS conflict content: Separation conflict

Example:
The father goes on a business trip. The
child experiences that for the first time
and doesn't understand that he is only
temporarily gone.

The one-time experience that
separations are not final and don't last
forever seems to be so dramatic, that
this kind of conflict usually occurs only
once.

PCL phase: Rash, etc.

Child
Child in reference to the
categorization of conflicts according
to the New Medicine
See: Partner

Chondroma
Term from the traditional medicine
Meaning: Cancer originating from
chondral tissue

According to the NM:
According to the NM, cancers originating
from chondral tissue can be attributed
to the mesoderm.

Cold, allergic
A SBS, which occurs due to a track and
not as a result of a DHS

See:
Head cold
SBS
Track
Conflict resolution

Cold nodule
See: Thyroid dysfunctions

Colon ascendens carcinoma
See: Large intestine cancer
Colon transversum carcinoma
See: Large intestine cancer
Colon carcinoma
See: Large intestine cancer

Common cold
See:
Head cold
Cough
Bronchitis
Influenza
Influenzal infection

Conflict classifications
Conflicts of "fear breathing down one's neck" – see: Glaucoma

Defilement conflict – see: Lupus, face eczema

Chunk conflicts – see: Palatal carcinoma, pituitary gland tumor, stomach cancer, thyroid dysfunctions, and bronchial cancer of the goblet cells in the bronchi

Refugee conflict – see: Gout, syndrome

Frontal fear conflict – see: Migraine

Conflict of "wanting to be seen" or "not wanting to be seen" – see: Inflammation of the lacrimal gland duct

Nasty, half-genital conflict – see: Ovarian cancer, prostrate cancer

Nasty, indigestible anger – see: Appendicitis

Identity conflict – see: Stomach ulcer

Conflict of "being unable to feed the family/children" – see: Pituitary gland tumor

Conflict of "wanting or not wanting to take in chunks of light" – inflammation of the iris

Conflict of being powerless – see: Thyroid dysfunctions

Conflict of threat to the territory – see: Asthma

Conflict of territory trouble – see: Stomach ulcer

Territory conflict, conflict of territory loss – see: Heart attack

Conflict of territory marking – see: Stress urinary incontinence, occlusion of the urethra

Fear due to shock – see: Asthma

Sexual conflict – see: Heart attack, uterine cancer

Stink conflict – head cold, inflammation of the sinuses

SWE (self-esteem conflicts) – see: Gout, varies, phlebitis, momma, hip joint pain, hand joint pain, foot joint pain, knee pain, shoulder pain, neck pain, pubic bone pain, skullcap pain, back pain, polyarthritis, lupus

Separation conflicts – see: Conjunctivitis, chicken pocks, lupus, neurodermatitis, soft tissue rheumatism, Alzheimer's

Conflict of loss – see: Ovarian cancer, endometrial cancer

Distorted perception – see: Irregular curvature of the cornea

Conflict mass
The conflict mass can be calculated from the product of conflict intensity and conflict duration.

However, being in constellation doesn't build up a lot of conflict mass.

In conflicts controlled by the old brain the conflict mass is proportional to the tumor size.

The conflict mass can possibly be reduced by taking baths. (See: Syndrome)

See also:
Conflict resolution
Downtransforming
Constellation
Track

Conflict resolution
Once the program is triggered only by accompanying tracks (smell, colour, material, etc.), as it were, but the actual conflict doesn't play a real role any longer, it is enough to become aware of that fact to stop the repetitive relapsing SBS forever.

It is more complicated if the conflict content as such still presents a danger, because it is current or occurs over and over again. Then, the individual must try to avoid experiencing the tracks, that is, the actual conflict content.

It is considered a great success, if the individual can develop some kind of a "calm/unaffected" attitude towards the original conflict content, although the danger is still present. The problem as

147

such doesn't touch the individual any more even though it is still present or it is possible to run into it again and again.

See also:
Downtransforming
Tracks
Conflict mass
Constellation

Conjunctivitis
See: Pinkeye

Conn's syndrome
Diagnoses of the traditional medicine: overproduction of the aldosterone due to an adenous tumor of the adrenal cortex. Further symptoms: High blood pressure, potassium deficiency, and nycturia

Possible cause according to the New Medicine:
See: Cushing's syndrome

Constellation
Schizophrenic constellation

If two SBSs are active and take place at the same time and their HH are located in both the right and the left brain hemisphere, the individual is in a state of schizophrenic constellation.

It means that either two DHSs struck each in the right and the left hemisphere, or a DHS has caused several conflicts, which caused one HH in each hemisphere.

If a constellation exists, there is more or less no or little buildup of conflict mass until one of the conflicts is resolved again. Hence, at least the resolution of the second conflict presents only a small risk because it is in constellation from the start. However, the first conflict should be also resolved soon as it will immediately start building up conflict mass again. In addition, the already existing conflict mass of the first conflict has to be considered when the second DHS occurs.

Some constellations lead to emotional- or mental disorders. If one of the conflicts is resolved, e.g., a depression is immediately eliminated. In that case it has to be considered that the resolved conflict now enters the healing phase while the unresolved is immediately building up conflict mass again. It is strongly recommended to resolve a

constellation with the help of a therapist as life-threatening complications can occur.

See also:
Conflict resolution
Downtransforming

Cortisone
The first agent found in the adrenal cortex of humans was named cortisone. It derives from cortex. Cortisone belongs to the group of glucocorticoids (sugar hormones), as they are able to increase the blood sugar level.

Cortisone is one the preliminary stage of the actual hormone, cortisol, and is only used as a keyword for laymen in reference to corticosteroids in general.

Synthetic cortisone versions are among others:
Prednisolon,
Methylprednisolone,
Betamethasone,
Dextamethasone,
Triamcinolone,
Paramethasone, and fludrocortisone.

A dehydrated version of the cortisone is prednisone, the effect of which approximates four times the effect of cortisone.

According to Dr. Hamer, cortisone is among the group of sympathycotonics that increase stress. It has an anti-inflammatory effect and stops tissue swelling by interrupting or alleviating the PCL phase.

Among other things, cortisone is used to reduce the brain edema during the repair- and healing phase, respectively, if complications can be expected from an excessive swelling.

A special application arises during the coping with the epileptoid - and healing crises, respectively. Provided the stress-inducing cortisone is applied at the right time and in the appropriate dose, it influences the depth of the healing phase. The cortisone works against the vagotony (gets the patient out of the dark whole in time) and helps to alleviate the epileptic crisis.

Attention! With syndrome, cortisone has the so-called paradox effect, because it intensifies the conflict active phase of

148

the kidney tubular-SBS (Meaningful Special Biological Program) and, thus, the buildup of excess fluid. As a second conflict is in the process of being resolved and the appropriate brain relay swells in the repair phase, it can lead to a particularly dangerous swelling in the brain; as well in the organ, for example, swelling of the liver.

In the New Medicine, cortisone is applied to alleviate life-threatening symptoms. It causes the edema in the brain to abate and, thus, reduces the organic symptoms as well, but prevents at the same time a complete healing.

The intake should always happen under the direction and the control of an experienced therapist!
No self-medication!
Important: Cortisone mustn't be discontinued abruptly, but the dose should be reduced gradually over several days or weeks.

See also: Epileptic crisis

Cough
See:
Bronchitis
Pneumonia
Lung cancer
Bronchial cancer
Bronchial cancer of the goblet cells in the bronchi
Asthma
Cystic fibrosis

Cushing's syndrome
DHS-conflict content: Conflict of "being thrown off the track", "having chosen the wrong path", or "having backed the wrong horse"

Example:
CA phase: Necrosis of the adrenal cortex, reduced cortisol expulsion resulting in "stressed fatigue", Waterhouse-Friedrichsen syndrome, Addison's syndrome (adrenal cortex insufficiency)

PCL phase: Filling of the necroses to the point of a fist-sized adrenal cortex cyst. Hardening of the cyst and overproduction of cortisol, Increased production of aldosterone, hirsutism, Cushing's syndrome

Germ layer: Mesoderm
Cerebral cortex hemisphere

Cystic fibrosis
See: Bronchial cancer of the goblet cells in the bronchi

Dementia
Old age dementia
See: Alzheimer's disease

DHS
Dirk Hamer syndrome
Named after Dr. Hamer's son, Dirk Hamer

A DHS is a shock that catches an individual completely off-guard (conflict shock); it meets three preconditions:
- severe (existential)
- highly acute–dramatic
- isolating

- The more importance the experiencing individuals attribute FOR THEMSELVES to the experience, the more severe is a DHS.
An event that the experiencing individuals don't interpret as important for their lives doesn't cause a DHS.
- The event surprised the individuals, so it caught them "on the wrong foot". They didn't anticipate it to happen. Hence, events that are anticipated don't cause a DHS either.

Experiencing the same event in a protected and safe environment also prevents the development of a DHS. The isolating aspect as such is also crucial, but not necessarily the period of time the individuals had to endure it on their own.

The DHS occurs simultaneously on three levels:
- in the psyche
- in the brain
- in the organ

The content of the DHS determines the location in the brain, the so-called Hamer Focus (HH; see: HH). The HH determines the affected organ and the processes there.

The so-called Meaningful Special Biological Program (SBS; see: SBS) starts directly with the DHS.

The same experienced conflict content of a DHS can nevertheless differ from individual to individual.

149

It is possible that in the moment of a DHS so-called tracks (see: Tracks) are developed; this can lead to repetitive relapses (e.g., allergies; see: Allergy).

See also the keywords:
HH
SBS
Tracks
Allergy
CA phase
PCL phase
Epileptic crisis
Conflict resolution
Conflict mass
Downtransforming

Diabetes
DHS-conflict content: Fear-disgust conflict, conflict of being reluctant

Handedness:
Right-handed woman:
Conflict 1 – fear-disgust conflict (hypoglycemia), conflict 2 – (because the female side of the brain is already blocked, now experienced in a male fashion, e.g.:) – being-reluctant conflict (hyperglycemia, diabetes)

Left-handed woman:
Conflict 1 – fear-disgust conflict (hyperglycemia, diabetes), conflict 2 - (because the male side of the brain is already blocked, experienced in a female fashion again, e.g.:) – another fear-disgust conflict (hypoglycemia)

Right-handed man:
Conflict 1 – being-reluctant conflict (hyperglycemia, diabetes), conflict 2 - (because the male side of the brain is blocked, now experienced in a female fashion, e.g.:) fear-disgust conflict (hypoglycemia)

Left-handed man:
Conflict 1 – being-reluctant conflict (hypoglycemia, diabetes), conflict 2 - (because the female side of the brain is blocked, experienced in a male fashion again, e.g.:) another being-reluctant conflict (hyperglycemia, diabetes)

Example:
Hypoglycemia
CA phase: Reduced glucagon production by the alpha islet cells, muscle trembling, increased feeling of hunger (to replenish sugar), weight gain, adiposity

PCL phase: Is not diagnosed as a disease; after the resolution of the conflict, sufficient glucagons are being produced again.

Diabetes
CA phase: Reduced function of the beta islet cells; insulin production decreases, blood sugar increases

PCL phase: (Regarding diabetes) – the beta islet cells produce insulin again; first excessively, which results in hypoglycemia (hypoglycemic shock, diabetic coma, but the production normalizes in the end.

Specific feature:
Type I diabetes: One brain relay active (Being-reluctant conflict), type II diabetes (adult onset diabetes): Two brain relays active, therefore conflicts in constellation (conflict of being reluctant and fear-disgust conflict)
Type II diabetes

See: diabetes
Type I diabetes

See: diabetes
Diabetic coma

See: Diabetes
Large intestine-TB

CA phase: Growing cauliflower-like compact tumors (adenocarcinoma)

PCL phase: Caseating, necrotisizing decomposition of the tumor through tumor mycosis fungoides, occasionally moderate bleeding or mycobacteria (large intestine-TB)

Germ layer: Endoderm
Hamer Focus in the brain:
Hamer Focus in the left lateral pons

Dirk Hamer syndrome
See: DHS
Named after Hamer's son, Dirk

Disseminated
Term from the traditional medicine
Meaning: Spreading of metastases through surgery

DNA
Deoxyribonucleic acid
Biochemical term;
Biochemical background: The DNA consists of...of the ribose.

The ribose is a sugar similar to regular sugar used in the kitchen. However, there is a certain location where the ribose lacks an oxygen atom, so it is "deoxidized" (oxidized=connected to an oxygen atom like iron oxide, aka rust). Thus, deoxyribo...

...of a phosphate
...of a base

Bases are small molecules, of which only four different kinds occur in the DNA:
Adenine
Guanine
Cytosine
Thymine

The sugar and the phosphate together are called nucleoside. If the base is added as well, it is referred to as a nucleotide. Several nucleotides combined cause the molecule to become "acidic" in nature in the chemical sense. Thus, ribonucleic acid.

The DNA strings, which developed that way, are today in every known living being. The units that are connected to threads are called "chromosomes". Humans have 46 chromosomes in the nucleus.

The DNA as a storage medium for information (the gene code or our genetic material):

The fact that only 4 different bases are used in the DNA could lead to the assumption that not very much can be achieved. However, a computer uses only TWO different pieces of information, namely "1" and "0", also called the binary code.

The DNA works very similar. The sequence of the 4 bases is crucial for the information that has to be stored. This sequence is "read" through different mechanisms (actually only chemical components like protein or sugar, which work together very well). Three bases at a time constitute the code for one amino acid. There are 21 amino acids that are important for mammals. In turn, the amino acids are combined to big molecules, the proteins. Their function depends, among other things, on the sequence of the amino acids, which is also determined by the DNA.

That means that these 4 building blocks are sufficient to cipher our entire genetic code.
In addition, the DNA also works extremely efficient by taking advantage of the following circumstance:

Of these 4 bases, only two match in a way that they can build a strong connection (hydrogen bridging). (Across from each other, not next to each other; phosphates and sugar are responsible for the connection from one nucleotide to another as a "chain".

"Guanine and cytosine" is the one pair (with three "bridges") and "adenine and thymine" is the other (with two "bridges").

That means that we don't have just one DNA string but two, which are mirrored against each other. However, the "mirror image" of a DNA sequence has necessarily a different base sequence, which, in turn, can be read and worked on. This way, we get double the amount of information.

That makes the DNA the simplest and yet the most effective storage medium on this planet.

See also: RNA

Downtransforming
The so-called downtransforming of a conflict becomes especially important if a conflict shouldn't be resolved any more because it lasted too long, or it was too intense, as a very vehement healing or even a fatal outcome has to be expected.

If the conflict has been downtransformed, the individual can also live with it until he or she is old and gray.

Downtransforming a conflict means that although the conflict has not been resolved, it still becomes less important for the individual. But the conflict remains lightly active.

It is the therapist's job to determine, when it is appropriate to resolve a conflict and when it is better to downtransform it.

See also:
Conflict resolution
Constellation

Ductal carcinoma in situ (DCIS)
Intraductal breast carcinoma
Mastitis

DHS conflict content: Separation conflict
("wanting/not wanting to be separated")

Example:
A mother worries about her son who
moves out from home, or she wants him
to finally move out

CA phase: Drawing in of the nipples;
mild, dragging pain

PCL phase: Swelling behind the nipples,
mastitis, (typical finding of the
traditional medicine)
Condition after the healing:
Microcalcification, (spatters of
calcification, milk that remained in the
breast)

Therapy: make the milk flow, "massage
out the milk"

See also: Breast cancer

Duodenal ulcer
See: Stomach ulcer

Ectoderm

This term refers to the categorization of
body tissue according to germ layers.
The following text was taken in its
original form from Dr. Hamer.

Quotation:
Ectoderm (outer germ layer)
Development situation:
Survival outside the safe ocean on land;
imminent threats; therefore, it was
necessary to develop organs that could
provide exact information about the
surroundings. Everything that was
allowed inside the body had to be
checked for its use, which made it
necessary to join forces with members
of the same kind.

Conflict situation:
Conflicts of admitting and eliminating,
that is, boundaries; conflicts of sensory
perception; conflicts of the contact with
other members of the species.

Organs that belong to the outer germ
layer:
All organs responsible for the connection
with the outside world:
- all sense organs

- the intima of the coronary arteries and
–veins, which developed from the
brachial archs

All access- and exit routes of the vital
organs:
- the liver (bile ducts)
- the pancreas
- the bronchi of the lungs
- the entrance and exit of the stomach,
etc.

All organs needed for the
communication or for the mutual setting
of boundaries:
- all external genitals
- the bladder
- the teeth
- the epidermis
- the muscles

Brain category:

The cerebral cortex
End of quotation

Source:
http//:www.pilhar.com/Hamer/NeuMed/
Kurzeinf/06Keimbl.html

Ectomy

Term from the traditional medicine;
meaning: surgical removal of an organ
(exception: resection [removing part of
the organ])

EK
EK=epileptic crisis
See: Epileptic crisis

Elbow pain
Rheumatism
DHS conflict content: SWE, not being
able to hit

Example:
CA phase: Bone osteolyses in this area,
anemia

PCL phase: Edema and expansion of the
periosteum, pain, recalcification,
leukemia, and joint rheumatism (in
traditional medicine often: arthritis)

The recalcification corresponds with the
diagnosis of the traditional medicine:
osteosarcoma

Germ layer: Mesoderm

See also: SWE

152

Embryology

The terms used in the New Medicine that relate to the germ layers originate from the science of embryology.

However, the terms are used with a different meaning in the New Medicine and the traditional medicine. While the traditional medicine classifies the different kinds of tissue in detail, the New Medicine mainly differentiates (rough classification):

Endoderm: Secretory/resorptive cells
Mesoderm: Connective/supporting tissue, muscles, etc.
Ectoderm: Squamous epithelium and sensitive, that is, nerve cells

While the traditional medicine associates the kinds of tissue with the individual organs, the New Medicine rather uses them to systemize the tissue **layers**.

One single organ can consist of all 3 types of tissue.

Endocarditis
See: Inflammation of the endocardium

Endocarditis
DHS conflict content: SWE regarding the performance of the heart

Example:
CA phase: Endothelial necroses, necroses of the heart valves

PCL phase: Endocarditis, endothelial calluses, heart valve alterations

Germ layer: Mesoderm

Endometrial cancer
DHS conflict content: A) a nasty, half-genital conflict (often with a man), or: B) a conflict of loss, especially grandmother/grandchild conflict

Example:
A) An older businesswoman finds out that an employee was caught with a minor. In order to get rid of him she has to pay him extensive compensation.

In general: Half-genital means that the emphasis of the conflict content is not on the purely genital area, but the topic occurs in the background.

CA phase: Compact tumor

PCL phase: Caseating decomposition with light bleeding (postmenopausal) or ejection with heavy bleeding (pre-menopausal)

Germ layer: Endoderm

See also:
Uterine cancer

Endometriosis
Also: Uterine catarrh

Endometrium
Uterine mucosa

Endometriosis is a condition where tissue similar to that of the endometrium can be found in locations it doesn't belong, for example, outside the uterus, or in locations of other mucosae, for instance, in the lung.

The traditional medicine characterizes this usually as "benign growth". The manifestations are manifold, from cysts to large areas. The tissue acts similar to the endometrium to the point of hormone-dependent monthly bleeding.

From the perspective of the New Medicine:
Conflict content: Always a nasty incident with a man

According to Dr. Hamer, it is not possible to have an endometriosis in the abdomen. The disease originates in the endometrium (too strong a constitution). Anatomically speaking, it is also impossible that such endometrium shreds can move from the uterus into the abdomen (or into the lung). If such "shreds" are found spread in the abdomen, they are cells of a burst ovarian cyst. These cells can continue to multiply for some time (up to 9 months after the CL). Then there are in fact small ovaries all over the abdomen. The CT of the brain confirms that is "only" an ovarian cyst. The relay for the endometrium stays "clean".

The real endometriosis that originates from the endometrium is "treated" with a conflict resolution (always a nasty incident with a man).
The New Medicine can't cure the wrongly diagnosed endometriosis (the things that float around in the

abdomen). Since the ovarian cyst is growing during the healing phase, it will remain even after the healing phase is completed (by and by the tissue will concentrate). If these "little lumps" bother the woman and cause problems, the only option is to have them surgically removed. The intake of hormones is tricky, because they can have side effects. Often women have more problems with taking hormones than without.

If "uterine tissue" has been removed from the lung, for example, it means that "shreds" of the ovarian cyst have been removed. Tissue identification (the rule of thumb in the traditional medicine): The histologist confirms the doctor's suspicion.

Endoderm
This term refers to the categorization of body tissue according to germ layers. The following text was taken in its original form from Dr. Hamer.

Quotation:
Endoderm (inner germ layer)
Development situation

Surviving and multiplying:
The first organisms were single-celled and on this stage of development they depended directly on their natural habitat, the ocean, and were in direct contact with it.
The multi-celled organisms further developed their survival organs from the same situation according to their archetypes from the inner germ layer.

Conflict situation:

Conflicts dealing with the "grasping of a chunk", for example, "not being able to grasp the chunk", or "not being able to swallow a chunk";
Fear of death conflicts
Existence conflicts
Nasty conflicts, e.g., nasty indigestible anger, nasty genital conflict, severe conflicts of loss

Organs of the inner germ layer:
All vital organs like the digestive organs, that is, the middle part of the stomach, the intestine without the rectum, a part of the liver, the lung, the prostate, the uterus without the cervix.

Affiliation in the brain:
The brain stem
End of quotation

Source:
http//:www.pilhar.com/Hamer/NeuMed/Kurzeinf/06Keimbl.html

See also: Ectoderm and mesoderm

Epi-crisis
See: Epileptic crisis

Epileptic crisis
Epileptic crisis, epileptoid crisis, epi-crisis, EC

The epileptic crisis is the lowest point of vagotony during the healing phase (PCL phase). Here, the brain edema is the largest and there is a possible danger at this point (e.g., a heart attack). Once the epileptic crisis is overcome, the patient is usually "out of the woods".

Emergency aid at home during the epileptic crisis:
Ice pack on the head (where the Hamer Focus is located, if known), elevating of the head or the upper body in bed, administering of glucose, honey, lemon juice. If possible, also walks in cool or cold air without a hat. No warmth, no direct sunlight on the head (not at all during the entire phase of vagotony!).
As a prescription:
Cortisone, where applicable; possibly other.
No cortisone in an active refugee conflict! (See: Cortisone)
Never administering of morphine in vagotony, it can result in death!
See also: Cortisone

Epileptoid crisis
See: epileptic crisis

Euthyroid
Euthyroid= normal production of thyroid hormones
See also:
Thyroid dysfunctions

Face eczema
DHS conflict content: Separation conflict or defilement conflict

Example:
A woman has a separation conflict because she is afraid her husband could leave her as he flirts with other women, or even cheats on her.

Or he makes her feel devalued; she feel like a "cleaning rug", as if she would get "nothing but dirt thrown into her face" (in regards to facial skin)

PCL phase: Red, swollen rash

See also:
Lupus

Fatigue, stressed
See: Cushing's syndrome

Finger joint problems
Rheumatism
DHS conflict content: SWE of the skillfulness

Example:
CA phase: Bone osteolyses in this area, anemia

PCL phase: Edema and expansion of the periosteum, pain, recalcification, leukemia, and joint rheumatism (in traditional medicine often: arthritis)

The recalcification corresponds with the diagnosis of the traditional medicine: osteosarcoma

Germ layer: Mesoderm
See also: SWE

Gastritis
See: Stomach ulcer

Germ layers
In the New Medicine, organs are associated with the biogenetically significant germ layers in regards to their categorization and progression. Biogenetically speaking, every germ layer corresponds to a specific part of the brain. In addition, the affiliation with a germ layer provides already information about the "type" of disease; the microbe, which will be active in the PCL phase; as well as the conflict content and also about the biological purpose (SBS). Most organs originate from only one germ layer, some, however from several germ layers.

Inner germ layer – endoderm
Attributed to the brain stem

The inner germ layer concerns the inner organs like the stomach, the intestine, liver, lungs, prostate, uterus, and the kidneys (kidney tubuli).

The conflict contents include e.g., the chunk conflicts, fear of death conflicts, existence conflicts, nasty indigestible anger, and severe conflicts of loss.

Events in the organ: Compact tumors

In the PCL phase active are: Fungi and particularly tuberculosis bacilli (mycobacteria amongst others)

Middle germ layer – mesoderm
Attributed to the cerebellum as well as the white matter of the cerebrum

The middle germ layer concerns organs like bones, cartilage, tendons, and hormone glands like the ovaries, the testicles, breast glands, adrenal glands, salivary gland, and further the blood vessels, blood- and lymph cells, lymphatic glands, the spleen, kidneys, sclera, as well as organ-covering membranes like the pleura and the pericardium.

Conflict contents are for example:
Collapse of self-esteem

Events in the organ: Compact tumors (cerebellum), necroses (white matter)

In the PCL phase active are:
Tuberculosis bacilli, other mycobacteria, and bacteria

Outer germ layer – ectoderm
Attributed to the cerebral cortex

The outer germ layer concerns organs like the sense organs, intima of the coronary arteries and –veins, liver- and bile duct, pancreas, bronchi, access routes of the stomach, etc., external genitals, bladder, teeth, skin, and muscles.

The conflict contents are conflicts dealing with boundaries, sensory perception, and contact with others, for example, separation conflict, conflict of territory marking, and fear-disgust conflict.

Events in the organ: Abscesses, function loss (e.g., diabetes), palsies

In the PCL phase active are: Viruses, bacteria

Goblet cells
Goblet cells of the bronchi

Intrabronchial remains of the old intestinal mucosa. Seen in the context of evolution, the intestinal mucosa germinated from the intestine and developed the lung alveoles.

Until today, the rare goblet cells of the bronchi, which produce the fluid in the bronchi, are the biogenetical-histological bridge links between the intestine and the alveoles.

Histological affiliation: endoderm
Hamer Focus (HH): brain stem

Gout
Acute gout attack
DHS conflict content: Constellation

Handedness:
Right-handed man: conflict 1 – SWE of athletic performance (bone osteolysis), conflict 2 – refugee conflict (kidney tubular carcinoma)

Example:
A youth was unsuccessful to score in a soccer game (athletic performance SWE). After he has just resolved this conflict, his father says, "When you turn 18 you have to move out." (refugee conflict). The right-handed teenager suffers a gout attack, e.g., in the left big toe.

See also:
SWE
Gout attack
Gout attack, acute

Glaucoma
Acute glaucoma
DHS conflict content: Fear breathing down one's neck (fear of the robber)

Example:
An item that is really important to a person and that this person wants to keep is in danger of being taken away by someone else.

Interestingly enough, in the traditional medicine they say that glaucoma develops due to strained eyes because of insufficient light". A typical example would be the intense search for the bottle of good wine in the dark basement. The strain and the bending down would often lead to the development of glaucoma.
The New Medicine's perspective: The cause is rather the good wine, that is, "the important item a person fears could have been taken or will be taken by someone else".

CA phase: Vitreous clouding, "tunnel vision phenomenon"

PCL phase: Acute glaucoma with increased eye pressure (=vitreous edema)

Germ layer: Ectoderm

GNM
GNM = Germanic New Medicine®
See also:
New Medicine
New Medicine according to Dr. Hamer
Germanic New Medicine®

Granulomatosis
See: Wegener's Granulomatosis

Hamer
Dr. med Ryke Geerd Hamer
Born in 1935, Ryke Geerd Hamer grew up in Friesia. After he finished his studies in medicine and theology, he worked in hospitals and as practicing physician.

In 1972, he became a specialist for internal medicine and worked as an internal specialist at the University of Tübingen. For years he was dealing with cancer patients.

Additionally, Dr. Hamer worked as an inventor. He owns different medical patents like, for example, a scalpel, which allows performing plastic surgery without bleeding (atraumatic).

In 1978, Dr. Hamer's son, Dirk, was shot on Corsica. Dirk died 3 months later after a leg amputation and 19 further surgeries at the university hospital of Heidelberg. This event changed Dr. Hamer's life. Shortly after his son's death Dr. Hamer developed testicular cancer.

From 1981 on he worked as head of the department in the cancer clinic associated with the university hospital of Munich. There, he thought about the possibility of his cancer being connected with the death of his son. He interviewed all the cancer patients in reference to potential existing shock experiences they had shortly before developing the disease and found those in every case.

In October 1981, when he wanted to make his discovery a subject of a medical discussion in the clinic, the management of the clinic told him to either renounce or leave the clinic.

He left the clinic, but not before he had searched all data of all the cancer patients and had recorded and secured the results, working day and night in his remaining time.

To date, according to his own statements, he checked his findings on the basis of 30,000 cases and all of them proved to be right.

Hamer Foci
See: HH

Hand joint pain
Rheumatism
DHS conflict content: SWE not getting a grip on the situation

Example:
CA phase: Bone osteolyses in this area, anemia

PCL phase: Edema and expansion of the periosteum, pain, recalcification, leukemia, and joint rheumatism (in traditional medicine often: arthritis)

The recalcification corresponds with the diagnosis of the traditional medicine: osteosarcoma

Germ layer: Mesoderm
See also: SWE

Head cold

DHS conflict content: Stink conflict "I am fed up to the back teeth with it."

Example:
Suddenly stepping outside where it is freezing cold; resolution, once the person is inside again where it is warm and comfortable; but also directly particular smells

CA phase: Nasal mucosa ulcers

PCL phase: Filling of the ulcers with new cells through swelling of the nasal mucosa with or without the participation of viruses; purulent head cold if inner bacterial mucosa parts are also affected

See also:

Inflammation of the paranasal sinuses, inflammation of the sinuses

Sense of smell, loss of

Healing phase of large intestine cancer

Decomposition of an adenocarcinoma in the intestine accompanied by mycobacteria; occasionally accompanied by moderate bleeding.

See also: Large intestine cancer
Large intestine cancer
Large intestine carcinoma =
Colon carcinoma, colon ascendens carcinoma, colon transversum carcinoma, colon descendens carcinoma

Biological conflict content:
Nasty, indigestible anger

Example:
Someone is accused of insurance fraud without good reason.

Heart attack
Angina pectoris
DHS conflict content: Territory conflict, threat-to-the-territory conflict (man), sexual conflict of "not being copulated with" (woman); watch constellation to some extent!

Handedness:
Right-handed woman:
Conflict 1 - sexual conflict of "not copulating" (cervical carcinoma, at the same time ulcer in the coronary veins), epileptic crisis after conflict 1:
Pulmonary embolism = acute right heart failure with right ventricular infarction; conflict 2 – territory conflict (coronary artery ulcer carcinoma), epileptic crisis after conflict 2, thus, only in constellation: Left ventricular infarction

Left-handed woman:
Conflict 1 – sexual conflict (coronary artery ulcer carcinoma), epileptic crisis after conflict 1: Left ventricular infarction; conflict 2 would be female side of the brain again, as male side is blocked, e.g., another sexual conflict (cervical carcinoma and coronary vein ulcer carcinoma); epileptic crisis after conflict 2: Right ventricular infarction (pulmonary embolism)

Right-handed man
Conflict 1 – territory conflict, (coronary artery ulcer carcinoma), epileptic crisis after conflict 1: left ventricular infarction; conflict 2 would be female side of the brain is blocked, e.g., another sexual conflict (seminal vesicle ulcer carcinoma and coronary vein ulcer carcinoma), epileptic crisis after conflict 2: Right ventricular infarction

Left-handed man
Conflict 1 – territory conflict (seminal vesicle ulcer carcinoma and coronary vein ulcer carcinoma), epileptic crisis after conflict 1: right ventricular infarction; conflict 2 – territory conflict (coronary artery ulcer carcinoma), epileptic crisis after conflict 2, that is, only in constellation: Left ventricular infarction

Attention: In addition to the handedness, the hormonal state also influences that side of the brain, in which the impact occurs. See: Handedness.

Example:
The territory or an essential part of the territory is lost. A territory can be: the company, the job, the house, car, the wife who runs away, etc. (man, territory conflict); a woman catches her husband and his lover in the act (woman, sexual conflict)

CA phase: Twinges in the left chest, angina pectoris

PCL phase: Angina pectoris, heart attack

Germ layer: Ectoderm

Characteristic: Generally, the heart attack is only noticed if the CA phase lasts longer than 3-4 months. However, if it lasts longer than 9 months in addition to average conflict intensity,

the patient is in danger of suffering a fatal heart attack during the epileptic crisis.

See also:
Uterine cancer
Sudden Cardiac Death (SCD)

Heart pain
See:
Angina pectoris
Heart attack

Hearing voices
Schizophrenia in terms of the traditional medicine

DHS conflict content: Double hearing conflict, thus, schizophrenic constellation. Hearing conflict in terms of a "speech tinnitus".

Example:
One (or both) hearing conflicts were triggered by words (instead of noises)

CA phase: Possibly tinnitus noises, but also the "hearing of voices"

PCL phase: Acute hearing loss; after a conflict resolution the schizophrenic constellation ends and the hearing of voices stops

Germ layer: Ectoderm

Characteristic: In an additional aggressive-biomanic constellation, the person firmly believes in an "order" the voices gave him or her. For example, many religious fanatics "hear voices" in a constellated hearing conflict plus aggressive-biomanic constellation.

See also:
Tinnitus
Acute hearing loss

Schizophrenia in terms of the traditional medicine

Paranoid schizophrenia
Paranoia

Heel bone pain
Rheumatism
DHS conflict content: SWE, "not being able to scrunch a situation"

Example:
CA phase: Bone osteolyses in this area, anemia

PCL phase: Edema and expansion of the periosteum, pain, recalcification, leukemia, and joint rheumatism (in the traditional medicine often diagnosed as arthritis)

The recalcification corresponds with the diagnosis of the traditional medicine: osteosarcoma

Germ layer: Mesoderm
See also: SWE

Hemoglobin
The red pigment in the blood

Hemorrhoids
Healing phase of a rectum carcinoma. If necessary, measures to help the swelling go down, otherwise unproblematic healing up.

See: Rectum carcinoma Ulcer

Handedness
In the New Medicine, it is important to know the handedness of a person, that is, whether he or she is left- or right-handed.
Some conflicts impact different brain areas depending on the handedness and can affect a different organ in each case. Only with organs controlled by the cerebellum is the handedness not important.

In addition to the handedness, the sex, whether male or female, is also important in determining the relevant brain areas as well as the organs. Equally important are hormonal changes due to taking the pill, age (climacterium), ovary radiation, hormone intake, etc. However, the hormonal situation is only relevant in regards to the consideration of the conflicts and the sequence of the impacts in the cerebral cortex.

The mother/child- and partner sides don't change however. They remain the way they are throughout a person's life.

But if a different brain area is affected (the so-called Hamer Focus, HH; see there), another organ will be affected based on that HH.

The handedness can be checked with different simple tests, e.g., the clap test (which hand is on top during clapping = handedness).

Hepatitis
DHS conflict content: Territory trouble conflict

Example:
The borders to the neighbouring territories are violated, so that the "neighbouring boss" can encroach. Often arguments about money.

PCL phase: Hepatitis with hepatitis A and B viruses or without (hepatitis non-A, non-B), danger of a liver coma immediately after the epileptic crisis, which is actually a brain coma. Therapy: Constant supply with glucose. Cortisone only in case of an emergency, or in combination with territory conflict (see: Heart attack).

Germ layer: Ectoderm

Characteristic: If the DHS conflict content is fear of starvation or fear of existence, the hepatitis is one possible form of the healing phase of a solitary liver carcinoma

HH
HH = Hamer Foci
Every brain relay has a certain connection with an organ and the HH in this location shows this reference as well. Dr. Hamer created a topography of the Hamer Foci of the brain. One single HH can also concern several organs, (several conflict impacts in the same moment). In turn, the location of the HH is determined by the conflict content of the DHS.

The Hamer Focus is visible in a CAT scan in both the CA phase and the PCL phase: In the CA phase it appears as "sharp concentric rings", which are often misinterpreted by traditional physicians as "ring artifacts"; in the PCL phase it appears as an edema, which is often misinterpreted as a brain tumor in the traditional medicine. The edema develops through accumulation of glia cells, which help to repair the HH, so that the defective brain relay will be fully functional again after the healing. An exception is the syndrome (a simultaneously active refugee conflict during the healing of another conflict), in which case excess fluid is being accumulated.

As the conflict is growing, so does the HH, and the correlating events in the organ are also progressing. In the CA phase, the concentric-ring configuration grows, and the HH grows in the PCL phase due to edema formation (accumulation of glia cells).

So, glioblastomas and such are no brain tumors but the condition of a HH in the healing phase. At the end of the healing phase the so-called "pee phase" takes place (increased urinating), in which the edema is being flushed out again.

See also:
DHS
SBS
CA phase
PCL phase
Epileptic crisis

Hip joint pain
Rheumatism
DHS conflict content: SWE "being unable to stand something"

Example:
A teacher is afraid of being attacked by parents during an uncomfortable conversation. She fears that instead of sticking to her conviction she will give in (in regards to the hip joint, being unable to stand something).

CA phase: Bone osteolyses

PCL phase: Recalcification, pain in the hip joints, (edema and expansion of the periosteum), leukemia, and joint rheumatism (in the traditional medicine often diagnosed as arthritis)

See also:
SWE

Hirsutism
See: Cushing's syndrome

Hoarseness
Conflict of threat to the territory, or conflict of fear due to shock depending on handedness and sex; for a description see under asthma.
See: Asthma

Hyperthyreosis
See: Thyroid dysfunctions

Hypoglycemia
See: Diabetes

Hypoglycemic shock
See: Diabetes

Hypothyreosis

See: Thyroid dysfunctions

Inflammation of the iris

DHS conflict content: Wanting or not wanting to take in chunks of light

Example:
A fortune, a job, etc. that seems within reach appears to be the possibility of realizing everything a person has dreamed of (extravagant lifestyle, etc.) and he or she desperately wants to have it now (wanting to take in chunks of light).

A child hears tires creaking and some noise. As it looks out of the window it sees an accident and recognizes the mother who is lying on the ground bleeding and severely injured. The child refuses to believe what it just saw (not wanting to take in the chunk of light). Incidentally, the noises of the accident could develop into a track.

PCL phase: Inflammation of the iris

Inflammation of the lacrimal canal

DHS conflict content: Conflict of "wanting to be seen" or "not wanting to be seen"

Example:
An analysis important for a person's business is overlooked, because other people push themselves forward, or interfere with their matters his or her matters (wanting to be seen).

A journalist desperately wants to ask a question, but he doesn't get noticed among all the other journalists (wanting to be seen).

CA phase: Ulcer formation in the lacrimal canal

PCL phase: Decomposition of the ulcer through bacteria or viruses with swelling of the mucosa, possibly blockage of the lacrimal canal (obstructed tear outflow)

Germ layer: Ectoderm

160

Inflammation of the paranasal sinuses
See: Head cold

Inflammation of the parotid gland
See: Mumps

Inflammation of the sinuses
See: Head cold

Inflammation of the tonsils
Tonsillitis

DHS conflict content: "Being unable to swallow a chunk" (because he or she can't – or doesn't want to; thus, having to spit out the chunk – or, also, wanting to but not allowed to)

Example:
An apartment a person would like to rent was rented to someone else. A child wants to spit out the spinach, but has to swallow it.

CA phase: Enlarged craggy tonsils (tonsillar hyperplasia, tonsillar hypertrophy)

PCL phase: Inflammation of the tonsils, purulent tonsillitis

Germ layer – endoderm, attributed to the brain stem

Influenza
Term from the traditional medicine

According to the traditional medicine, clinical pictures that match a special type, which is defined by the symptoms, are referred to as "influenza" or "influenzal infection".

These are symptoms like a head cold, a cough, (diseases of the mucous membrane), joint pain or overall weakness of the body. It is assumed, that viruses are the cause for the condition.
Explanation according to the NM after Dr. Hamer: The so-called influenza symptoms are also to be interpreted according to the five laws of nature. Every symptom corresponds with a Hamer Focus in the brain and originates in an associated conflict.

As the traditional medicine doesn't provide a precise definition or symptom affiliation, it is difficult to come up with a categorization.

For example, a combination of a resolved self-esteem conflict (in the healing phase light case of leukemia, swollen lymph nodes, fatigue, and joint pain) and a conflict of threat to the territory, which was resolved (in the healing phase bronchitis), can be diagnosed as influenza.

Influenzal symptoms are always the healing phase (PCL phase).

See also:
Bronchitis
Cough
Head cold
Asthma
SWE
Pneumonia

Influenzal infection
See: Influenza

Intraductal breast carcinoma
See: Mamma carcinoma

Intrahepatic bile duct ulcer
A possible form of healing phase of a solitary liver carcinoma

Irregular curvature of the cornea
See: Astigmatism
DHS conflict content: Distorted perception

Example:
A father abuses his child, but the child doesn't integrate this misbevaviour in its overall consideration of the father as a person.
The father can't or mustn't be seen for the person he really is, with all his good and bad sides.

Jaundice
See: Hepatitis

Joint rheumatism
See: SWE
Knee pain
Foot joint pain
Hand joint pain
Back pain, etc.

Knee pain
DHS conflict content: SWE of athletic performance

CA phase: Bone osteolyses in this area

PCL phase: Edema and expansion of the periosteum, pain, recalcification, leukemia, and joint rheumatism (in the traditional medicine often diagnosed as arthritis)

The recalcification corresponds with the diagnosis of the traditional medicine: osteosarcoma

Germ layer: Mesoderm
See also: SWE

Laryngeal cancer
Conflict of threat to the territory or conflict of fear due to shock, depending on handedness and sex
See: Asthma

Lid inflammation
See: Pinkeye

Lid margin inflammation
See: Pinkeye

Liver cirrhosis

One possible form of healing phase of the solitary liver carcinoma

Leukemia
Leukemia is the healing phase of a SWE, the PCL phase of a so-called bone cancer. Leukemia possibly causes severe brain symptoms (large edema of the HH); thus, seek treatment of a therapist of the New Medicine

DHS conflict content: SWE, see also under the respective classifications, e.g., knee joint, back, etc.

Example:
CA phase: Bone osteolyses in this area, anemia

PCL phase: Edema and expansion of the periosteum, pain, recalcification, leukemia, and joint rheumatism (in the traditional medicine often diagnosed as arthritis)

The recalcification corresponds with the diagnosis of the traditional medicine: osteosarcoma

Germ layer: Mesoderm
See also: SWE

Liver tuberculosis (liver TB)

One possible form of healing phase of the solitary liver carcinoma

Lung cancer

DHS conflict content: Fear-of-death conflict

Example:
Diagnosis of a "deadly disease" by a doctor

CA phase: Lung tumors / lung nodules

PCL phase: Caseating through mycobacteria; if not existent, encapsulation

Germ layer: Endoderm

See also:
Bronchial cancer of the goblet cells in the bronchi
Bronchial cancer

Lupus
Lupus erythematosus (SLE or lupus)

DHS conflict content: Facial skin affected = separation conflict or defilement conflict; hip joint affected = SWE (collapse of self-esteem) "being unable to stand something"; other organs = see there; possibly equivalent. They are individual specific conflicts in each case!

Example:
A woman has a separation conflict because she is afraid her husband could leave her as he flirts with other women, or even cheats on her. Or he makes her feel devalued; she feel like a "cleaning rug", as if she would get "nothing but dirt thrown into her face" (in regards to facial skin)

A teacher is afraid of being attacked by parents during an uncomfortable conversation. She fears that instead of sticking to her conviction she will give in (in regards to the hip joint, being unable to stand something).

PCL phase: In regard to the face, lupus nodules but also red, swollen rash; in regard to the hip joint, pain in the hip joints.

Germ layer: Different germ layers, depending on the conflict and the affected organ.
See also under germ layers
See also:
Face eczema
Hip joint pain

Lupus erythematosus
See: Lupus

Lymph nodes, swollen
DHS conflict content: Mild localized SWE

PCL phase: Swollen lymph nodes

Malignant
Often in connection with melanoma

Malignant
Malignant cells:
Definition according to SM:

- don't have distinct differentiations or outlines
- grow very fast
- uncontrolled growth (grow into "healthy" tissue)
- destroy surrounding tissue
- exceed histological borders ("limitless growth")
- redevelop after their removal
- metastatizing
- are not mature cells

"Malignant cells" form "malignant tumors",
e.g., Willms tumor, chest tumor, intestine tumor, etc.

According to Dr. Hamer's NM, "malignant tumors" rather correspond with the tumors controlled by the cerebellum (inner germ layer = "endoderm" or middle germ layer – mesoderm) in the CA phase (conflict active phase).

In this phase, the "tumor" still fulfills its biological special task and, thus, actively continues to grow.

The "metastasis" and the growth beyond the histological borders can be attributed to additional SBS and/or to consequent conflicts. Often connected with the cancer diagnosis (see: Lung cancer).

In this phase, different tumors secure their supply by building connections to the surrounding tissue and, thus, increase their blood circulation.
This behaviour is interpreted as "uncontrolled growth", which is misleading, because the growth doesn't occur uncontrolled but is subject to the rules of the SBS.

The appearance of a "malignant tumor" changes in the course of the development (aggravation or resolution of the conflict).
Example: "Willms tumor"
Other examples of "malignant cancer growth" are the tumors of the ectoderm (controlled by the cerebral cortex). If recognized as such in the CA phase, these "tumors" are so-called "ulcera", that is, "wholes" (cell degradation).

Among others, lung cancer and osteolysis (porous bones) belong to this group.
See also:
Benign
Metastasis
Cancer

Mamma carcinoma
See:
Breast cancer
Ductal carcinoma in situ (DCIS)
Ductal mamma carcinoma
Intraductal breast carcinoma
Mastitis
Mammary gland cancer

Mammary gland cancer
See: Breast cancer

Mastitis
See: Ductal carcinoma in situ (DCIS)

Measles
DHS conflict content: "I am fed up to the back teeth with it"-conflict
In addition: Conflict of "being unable to smell", "I am sick of that", "being unable to express things". The conflict affects the oral cavity and the sinuses.

PCL phase: Measles with rash, etc.

Melanoma
Malignant melanoma
Amelanotic melanoma

DHS conflict content: Defilement conflict, conflict of feeling hurt or scarred, e.g., by amputations, scars, wrinkles, but also by verbal insults or real defilement

Example:
Melanoma at scarred spots that are perceived defacing; melanoma at other body parts that create a conflict, as they are perceived as unattractive; melanoma as a result of insult or verbal attack that is felt at this particular part of the body ("It hit me like an arrow between the shoulders.")

CA phase: Melanoma is growing either compact, including a mole, or without pigment (amelanotic melanoma)

PCL phase: Smelly, caseating and necrotizing decomposition through mycobacteria or bacteria; only if the squamous epithelium covering it is open further cell division will stop.

Germ layer: Mesoderm, right hemisphere of the cerebellum

Mesoderm
This term refers to the categorization of body tissue according to germ layers. The following text was taken in its original form from Dr. Hamer.

Quotation:
Mesoderm (middle germ layer)
Development situation:

Protozoa developed into metazoa. They distance themselves from the ocean through a membrane. Thus, it is necessary to develop a fluid similar to the ocean water as well as a system of rules inside the united cell structure in order to sustain this emulated ocean water at all times. In the beginning, that is the task of the hormones. Then, nerve fibers develop from hormone streams that are always alike. To guarantee the living being the freedom to move, it needed movement organs.

Conflict situations:
Conflicts of adaptation, coordination, vulnerability and the ability to move
Organs belonging to the middle germ layer:

- skeleton: All of the bones, cartilage tissue, tendons,
- skeleton-, intestine-, and heart muscles
- hormone-producing glands like the ovaries, testicles, breast glands, and adrenal glands
- blood vessels, blood cells, lymph cells, lymphatic glands, spleen, kidneys
- sclera,
- all organ-covering membranes like the pleura and the pericardium

Brain category:
The body parts mentioned above are controlled by three different brain parts according to their history of development: The membranes are controlled by the cerebellum, the other parts by either the midbrain or the white matter of the cerebrum.
End of quotation

Source:
http//:www.pilhar.com/Hamer/NeuMed/Kurzeinf/06Keimbl.html

See also: Endoderm and ectoderm

Metastasis
From the perspective of the traditional medicine:

If, after the detection of one (malignant) cancer, another cancer is detected in the body of a patient, it can be assumed that the first one has "spread". Presumably, over time, further metastases will be found in the body of the patient, also originating from the first detected cancer. If the spreading can't be stopped using therapeutic methods (surgery, chemotherapy, radiation treatment), the patient is considered "untreatable".

The "spreading" can be triggered by just one single degenerated cell that was overlooked during surgery.

Therefore it is essential to detect the cancer as soon as possible by means of regular preventive medical checkups, and to start as soon as possible after surgery with a prophylactic therapy (chemotherapy, radiation treatment). The risk of metastases in women can be further reduced by giving them hormone supplements.

According to Dr. Hamer's New Medicine, "metastases" don't exist.

So far, every detected "metastasis" analyzed according to the New Medicine (if known) could be related to an associated HH as well as to a conflict content (with SBS).

For example, lung cancer, which is the most common secondary cancer, can be related to a fear of death conflict (with SBS) and very often occurs shortly after the patient received the cancer diagnosis.

See also:
Benign
Malignant
Cancer

Metastases
See: Metastasis

Migraine
DHS conflict content: Frontal fear conflict, "What will be in store for me?"

Example:
A student is notified that, in order to evaluate his grade point average, he alone has to take a test the very next day about the subject matter of the entire year. He is scared and worries: What will be in store for me?"

In general: Not being able to assess an impending situation in terms of how well it can be mastered, how it will proceed, and what the outcome will be.

PCL phase: Migraine attack
See also:
Panic attack

Mononucleosis
DHS conflict content: Generalized SWE

PCL phase: Mononucleosis

MS
MS = multiple sclerosis
See: Multiple sclerosis

Multiple sclerosis
(Palsy of the motor- and sensory nerves

DHS conflict content:
Extremities: A) arms: Unable to fend off or hold on to something; B) legs: Conflict of "being unable to escape or keep up"; also: "being at a loss";

C) Back- and shoulder muscles: conflict of "being unable to evade", secondary conflict in schizophrenic constellation: conflict of "being unable to ever walk again".
As well, these conflicts are often accompanied by a SWE.

Example:
Conflict of the motor nerves: A little girl suffered an enormous DHS when vaccinated against smallpox paravertebrally between the shoulder blades. Shortly after, all four of her extremities were paralyzed.

The doctors wrongly assumed a tumor in the vertebral canal, that is, an incomplete paraplegia. Thus, the conflict was kept active, as the doctors constantly manipulated the same spot. There is a great danger of a secondary conflict and, with it, a schizophrenic constellation because of the shock of the diagnosis, telling her that she is never going to walk again.

The clinical picture of MS also results from alternating CA- and CL- or PCL phases. As soon as the PCL phase occurs, it is accompanied by symptoms that, without the knowledge about the two phases of a disease, are interpreted as a "worsening" or just as "abnormal", and that can trigger a new SBS in the affected person. Due to the new SBS the PCL phase ends, which causes the affected person into thinking that his or her condition is "improving" because the symptoms abate. This cycle can repeat itself until it gives the impression of a chronic disease.

CA phase: Palsy, muscular atrophy

PCL phase: Resolution of palsy symptoms; epileptic crisis in a conflict involving motor nerves: seizure.

Germ layer: Ectoderm and mesoderm

See also:
Stroke
Parkinson's disease

Mumps
DHS conflict content of "being unable, being not allowed to, or not wanting to eat" (insalivate)

CA phase: Parotid gland ulcers, which often go unnoticed (dragging pain)

PCL phase: Mumps with or without the parotitis virus

Germ layer: Ectoderm, cerebrum hemisphere

Mutagen
Changes genetic material
See also: Carcinogen

Myoma
Uterine muscle cancer

DHS conflict content: SWE conflict of "not being pregnant"

CA phase: Necroses

PCL phase: Myoma

Germ layer: Mesoderm
See also: Uterine cancer

Myxedema
See: Thyroid dysfunctions

Nasopharyngeal adenoids
See: Adenoids

Natural laws
The five biological laws according to Dr. Hamer

First biological law:
The Iron Rule of Cancer
There are three criteria that have to be existent before the first biological law is fulfilled:

First criterion
Every cancer- or cancer-equivalent disease originates from a DHS, e.g., a very severe (existential),
highly acute-dramatic, and
isolating shock.
The experience of the shock conflict is simultaneous or virtually simultaneous on all three levels:

in the psyche
in the brain
in the organ

Second criterion
The conflict content determines in the moment of the DHS the location of the Hamer Focus in the brain as well as the corresponding location of the cancer- or cancer-equivalent disease in the organ.

Third criterion

The conflict development corresponds to a specific development of the Hamer Focus in the brain and a very specific development of a cancer- or cancer-equivalent disease in the organ.

Second biological law

The law of the two phases of all diseases (provided that there is a conflict resolution).

In the past, the traditional medicine defined several "cold diseases" and also several "hot diseases".

The "cold diseases" were those, during which the patients had cold outer skin and cold extremities, had constant stress, lost weight, and had problems to fall asleep or sleep through the night like for example cancer, MS, angina pectoris, neurodermatitis, diabetes, mental- or emotional disorders, etc.

The other kind of "diseases" were those the traditional medicine ranks among all so-called infectious diseases, also rheumatic diseases, allergies and dermatitises, respectively.

That is not exactly right. These "cold and hot diseases" weren't diseases at all but one of two phases of a disease, respectively: The cold stage is always the first phase, and the hot stage is the second.

Third biological law

The ontogenetic system of tumors and cancer-equivalent diseases

The ontogenetic system categorizes all so-called diseases according to their germ layer affiliation, that is, the inner-, the middle-, and the outer germ layer, which form as early as the beginning of the embryo's development.

Not only can every cell and every organ of the body be attributed to more than one of these germ layers, but each of

166

these layers have specific parts of the brain and also histological formations biogenetically belonging to them.

Furthermore, organs controlled by the cerebrum and those controlled by the old brain act inversely proportional to each other regarding cell multiplication and cell meltdown during the conflict active- and the healing phase.

Fourth biological law

The ontogenetic system of microbes

Without exception, every germ layer-related organ group has in the healing phase specific germ layer-related microbes. The microbes are not the cause of the healing symptoms but only the optimizers.

Fifth biological law

The biological meaning of each special program of nature

This law completely reverses the previous understanding of a disease.

The disease as such in the traditional sense doesn't exist any longer. All so-called "diseases" have a biological meaning, which hasn't been realized until now.

All diseases are caused by special programs that help us to survive and have been anchored in our brain from time immemorial. Thus, these meaningful special biological programs (SBS) are the perfect solution of our brain, the "last possibility to survive".

The individual SBSs are further explained in the "Scientific Table of the New Medicine".

Neck pain
Cervical spine

DHS conflict content: SWE in the intellectual area (injustice, feeling of being bound, strife, etc.)

Example:
"Stress" and devaluation in the workplace, which results in neck pain every evening

CA phase: Bone osteolyses in this area, anemia

PCL phase: Edema and expansion of the periosteum, pain, recalcification, and leukemia

Germ layer: Mesoderm
See also: SWE

New Medicine

The New Medicine, also called Germanic New Medicine since recently, was developed by Dr. Ryke Geerd Hamer after he had discovered several biological laws.

Neurodermatitis

DHS conflict content: Separation conflict, wanting to hold on to (extremity insides) or fend off someone (extremity outsides, etc.)

Example:
A man has an affair and doesn't touch his wife any longer. She is afraid of a separation and also misses the physical contact.

Occurrence in the palm of the hands and at the insides of the arms: Wanting to hold on (to the husband)

Occurrence at the outsides of the arms: Wanting to fend off (the opponent, but also the husband who hurt the wife after all), etc.

With the eczema occurring during the healing phase, there is an increased danger of relapse due to the husband's withholding of physical attention because of the woman's repulsive appearance.

Principally, we have a similar situation with children and their parents. With their desire to become independent of their parents usually arising during puberty, children often don't experience any or only few relapses from that time on.

CA phase: Somewhat rougher and more non-sensitive skin, mostly unnoticed

PCL phase: Eczema, exanthema, etc., the skin irritations are red, swollen, and itchy

167

NM
See: New Medicine

Obesity
See: Diabetes
Syndrome

Occlusion of the urethra
Stress urinary incontinence
DHS conflict content: Conflict of territory
marking

Example:
Not being able to mark the territory

CA phase: Spasm and ulcer
development

PCL phase: Swelling during healing;
remedy: bladder catheter until
symptoms abate

Germ layer: Ectoderm

Old Age Dementia
See: Alzheimer's

Oral thrush

See: Aphthous oral infection

Osteosarcoma

See: Organ categorization under SWE or
leukemia

Otitis of the middle ear
Eustachian tube carcinoma (between
mouth and middle ear)

Biological conflict content: "Being unable
to hear, absorb", or "grasp" an
important, necessary piece of
information or chunks of things that
have been said; also, wanting to get rid
of a piece of information or not wanting
to hear it.

Example:
A little girl who doesn't want to hear
about having to go to bed while her
older siblings can do the most exciting
things.

Hamer Focus in the brain: HH in the
right dorsal brain stem (pons)

Germ layer: Endoderm

CA phase: The Eustachian tube suffers
an obstruction due to the compact-
growing tumor.

Consequence: Drawn-in ear drum due to
lacking ventilation and bad hearing

PCL phase: Smelly caseation that
discharges into the mouth as well as
into the middle ear, faking an ear
infection (otitis media) unless the
mucous membrane of the middle ear
itself is also affected.

Ovarian cancer
DHS conflict content: Conflict of loss due
to death or leaving

Example:
A mother dies in the hospital and the
daughter feels guilty because she hasn't
visited her in a while. Without a "guilty
conscience" there is no conflict most of
the time.

CA phase: Necrosis

PCL phase: Cyst filled with fluid that
indurates, that is, the cyst hardens and
develops the tumor with supply
branches in the surrounding tissue. After
that, it encapsulates.
Surgery indicated only if it is
mechanically interrupting. This former
ovarian cyst has a rejuvenating effect,
because it produces a lot of estrogen.

Germ layer: Endoderm

See also:
Uterine cancer
Ovarian cyst
Ovarian cyst

See:
Ovarian cancer
Endometriosis
Fallopian tube cancer
Fallopian tube cancer

DHS conflict content: A nasty half-
genital conflict, mostly with a male
person

Example:
An older businesswoman finds out that
an employee was caught with a minor.
In order to get rid of him she has to pay
him extensive compensation.

In general: Half-genital means that the
emphasis of the conflict content is not
on the purely genital area, but the topic
occurs in the background.

CA phase: Compact tumor with regularly blocked fallopian tubes

PCL phase: Caseating decomposition through fungi and mycobacteria

Germ layer: Endoderm

See also:
Uterine cancer

Overweight
See: Diabetes
Syndrome

Palatal carcinoma
DHS conflict content: "Chunk already grasped but not being able to swallow it"

Example:
A lottery player expects a lottery win because his numbers were drawn. But without his knowledge his ticket wasn't handed in.

A worried mother expects a call from her child, which in on vacation, on a certain day, but the child only calls two days later.

CA phase: Cell multiplication, palatal tumor

PCL phase: Tumor decomposition through fungi and mycobacteria

Germ layer: Endoderm

Palliative medicine
According to the definition of the German Association of Palliative Medicine, palliative medicine is the treatment of patients who suffer from an incurable, progressive, and well-advanced disease and have a limited life expectancy; the main goal of the supportive care is the quality of life. Not the prolonging of the time a patient has left at all costs but the quality of life, that is, the wishes, goals, and the condition of the patient are the focus of the treatment.

Panic

See: Panic attacks

Panic attacks

Constellation of frontal fear conflict and conflict of "fear breathing down one's neck", both in their CA phase

Paranoia
See: Hearing voices

Paranoid schizophrenia
See:
Hearing voices
Tinnitus

Parkinson's
Parkinson's disease

The healing of a palsy of the motor nerves that never comes to a stop due to small relapses (the so-called hanging healing).

The Parkinson tremor is a form of healing, more specifically, a healing of a motor conflict of the motor nerves of the hand muscles.

See also: Multiple sclerosis

Parotitis
See: Mumps

Partner
According to the conflict categorization of the New Medicine, a partner is everyone except a person's own mother or a person's own child.

However, in specific cases other people are perceived as a mother or as a child as well, e.g., nurses for the elderly could consider the people they care for their children, or an older friend could be considered a mother.

PCL phase
PCL phase = conflict resolved phase (healing phase)

In the moment of the conflict resolution a person switches from being in the CA phase (conflict active phase) to being in the PCL phase. The CL phase is characterized by warm to hot hands (and feet), increasing appetite, fatigue and weakness (vagotony).

Also, the epileptic crisis (see: epileptic crisis), which could possibly take a critical course, takes place during the PCL phase.

In the PCL phase, the application of morphine is particularly risky and can lead to a person's death because it reinforces the vagotony.

See also:
CA phase
SBS
DHS
PCR

Pinkeye
DHS conflict content: separation conflict, to have lost sight of someone

Example: For the first time, the child goes on vacation alone and, for the first time, the parents don't see it every day any more

CA phase: Abscesses on the conjunctiva (also lid margin, lid)

PCL phase: Healing of the abscesses through bacteria or viruses, (conjunctivitis, lid margin inflammation, lid inflammation)

Germ layer: Ectoderm
See also:
Lid margin inflammation
Lid inflammation

Pituitary gland cancer
See also differentiation toward" brain tumor
DHS conflict content: A) "being unable to grasp the chunk", because the individual is too small, or B) conflict of being unable to feed the child and the family respectively

Example:
A man loses his job and can't find a new one; less money is available but he still continues to pursue his hobbies, which are now too expensive, and there is barely enough money to buy groceries. (For instance, the conflict is experienced by the wife/mother who worries about how to feed the family.)

CA phase: A) pituitary gland tumor with excretion of growth hormones. Consequences are: In children: growth; in adults: Acromegaly. B) Pituitary gland tumor with increased excretion of prolactin. Consequence is increased lactation.

PCL phase: Decomposition of the tumor (caseation) through fungi and mycobacteria.

Germ layer: Endoderm

Pneumonia
Epileptic crisis of the bronchial carcinoma
See:
Bronchial cancer
Bronchitis
Asthma

For differentiation:
Lung cancer
Bronchial cancer of the goblet cells in the bronchi

Polyarthritis
DHS conflict content: SWE regarding several joints; there are different individual conflicts: Conflict of "being unable to stand something", SWE of skillfulness, SWE of athletic performance, and others

CA phase: Bone osteolyses in different areas

PCL phase: Edema and expansion of the periosteum, pain, recalcification, leukemia, and joint rheumatism (in the traditional medicine often diagnosed as arthritis, here: polyarthritis)

The recalcification corresponds with the diagnosis of the traditional medicine: Osteosarcoma

Germ layer: Mesoderm

See the different individual conflicts under: SWE

Polymerase chain reaction (PCR)
A term from biotechnology; meaning: The chaining of DNA building blocks (nucleotides) on the basis of a model performed by the enzyme "polymerase". The PCR can be imagined like a kind of "DNA copier".

Application:
Whenever the DNA- or RNA sample is too small to analyze, or just a specific segment of the original is to be copied

The PCR is often mentioned as RT-PCR (reverse transcriptase PCR) in connection with HIV tests.

The PCR's principle:
A piece of double-stranded DNA serves as the "template". It has to be heated (95°C) in order to separate the strands, so that the enzyme polymerase can bind to the individual strands. In addition to the DNA and the enzyme, there are also individual nucleotides in the vial as well as so-called "primers".

The primers are also pieces of the DNA. They determine which DNA fragment is copied. Therefore, it is important that the experimenter knows exactly the composition and the sequence of the nucleotides of the primers, respectively. Normally they are produced especially for the respective use.

The primers fit only at a very specific location of the DNA and attach themselves there. The enzyme polymerase uses this beginning and extends it. Thus, a double-stranded DNA forms again, which is again separated into two strands by using heat, which, then, serve as a template of their own.

Depending on how often the temperature is raised and lowered again, a higher or lower number of the relevant DNA fragment is created.

Variation:
If the original material is RNA instead of DNA, the polymerase is unable to recognize the material and, consequently, to copy it. Therefore, another enzyme called the "reverse transcriptase" is used. It recognizes the RNA and produces copies from DNA.

Example:
The traditional medicine, especially the HIV tests (HIV is a retro virus, the genetic material of which consists of RNA, not DNA) assumes that the human body doesn't have the enzyme "reverse transcriptase".

So, they take the blood sample of a person as a template for the RT-PCR and DON'T add the enzyme. If, subsequently, the existence of DNA can be proven, the enzyme "reverse transcriptase" has to have been in the sample.

That is considered evidence for the existence of a HIV virus in the body and, thus, also as a "positive AIDS test", because traditional practitioners wrongly assume that the existence of the virus is synonymous with the clinical picture known as "AIDS".

Besides, the problem with this assumption is that there can be many other causes for the existence of "reverse transcriptase" in the blood as well. So, this evidence is not clear.

Prostrate cancer
DHS conflict content: Nasty, half-genital conflict

Explanation: The emphasis is not on the genital topic, but it occurs in the background.

Typical examples:

- the favourite daughter sues his father for financial support or early assess to her inheritance,

- the only daughter is delinquent or addicted to drugs,

- a man catches his wife/lover with a younger lover in the act,

- during a divorce very nasty things are brought to light,

- an older man is left by his younger girlfriend for a younger man

CA phase: Compact tumor, possibly restricted urinary flow (decreased urinary stream), no pain

PCL phase: Decomposition of the tumor through mycobacteria, no pain, urine is smelly and cloudy, possibly with traces of blood. If severe flow restriction: Catheter for the duration of the healing phase. Otherwise the healing is unproblematic, no danger of becoming impotent.

In case no mycobacteria are existent, the urine outflow returns back to normal nonetheless, because the swelling goes down. However, in rare cases surgery is necessary if the tumor, which is not being decomposed, puts too much pressure on the urethra.

Germ layer: Endoderm

Psoriasis
Simultaneous occurrence of both an active and a resolved separation conflict overlapping on one or several skin areas, which causes the scaling.

See also: Neurodermatitis

Pubic bone pain
DHS conflict content: Sexual SWE

CA phase: Bone osteolyses in this area, anemia

PCL phase: Edema and expansion of the periosteum, pain, recalcification, and leukemia

Germ layer: Mesoderm
See also: SWE

Pulmonary embolism
See: Cervical cancer, heart attack

Rectum carcinoma
See:
Stomach ulcer
Hemorrhoids

Relapse
Recurring

In the New Medicine the term "relapse" describes the re-occurring of a conflict and the re-occurring of a SBS, respectively.

See also: Tracks

Remission
Restoration, recovery

Rheumatism

See:
SWE
Back pain
Foot joint pain
Hand joint pain
Shoulder pain
Knee pain, etc.

RNA
Ribonucleic acid

RNA is very similar to DNA. However, there are two differences:

RNA uses ribose (not oxidized) as sugar.

RNA uses the base "uracil" instead of "thymine".

Therefore, RNA is perishable and normally decomposes within a few minutes. The organism uses RNA as a kind of "working copy" of the long-living DNA, for example in the production of proteins.

If a certain protein is to be produced, a RNA copy of the relevant DNA stretch is created first. The copy is processed a little further before it is transferred to the "ribosomes", which are the protein factories.

Some viruses have RNA instead of DNA as their genetic material, but they seem to manage quite well.

See also: DNA

SBS
SBS = Meaningful Special Biological Program

The SBS begins in the moment of the DHS, as the DHS strikes simultaneously in the psyche, the brain, and the organ.

The SBS is the alteration in the organ controlled by the Hamer Focus (HH). There are two phases: The conflict active phase (CA phase; see there) is characterized by sympathicotony; the individual is under "constant stress". Cold hands and feet and lack of appetite are the symptoms. The thoughts circle constantly around the conflict.

The relevant organ shows either cell growth or cell decomposition (necrosis), depending on the respective germ layer (see: Germ layers).

Is the patient able to resolve the conflict, he immediately enters the conflict resolved or healing phase (PCL phase; see there), which is characterized by warm hands; the patient is in vagotony, thus, rather tired and weak and his or her appetite increases. The possibly critical climax of the healing phase is the epileptic or epileptoid crisis (see: Epileptic crisis).

Now, cell growth and cell decomposition is taking place again. The cell decomposition occurs through fungi, mycobacteria (TB), bacteria, or viruses. If they are not existent, the tumors encapsulate. "Cancer tumors" (in the traditional sense) immediately stop growing and "inflammations" (in the traditional sense) develop immediately.

It is important to know that the New Medicine doesn't distinguish between benign and malignant tumors. The term cancer is referring here to the events at the organ level in general. Diseases that aren't cancer in the traditional sense are considered "cancer equivalent".

172

Hence, in the New Medicine all so-called diseases are referred to as "cancer".

The program is called meaningful special biological program because there is or once was a benefit behind it for the individual (in humans often only in the figurative sense). Cell multiplication, for example, is supposed to accomplish an increased capacity of the organ.

See also:
Germ layers
HH
CA phase
PCL phase
DHS
Epileptic crisis

Schizophrenia
(In the sense of the traditional medicine)
See: Hearing voices

Sense of smell, loss of
Loss of sense of smell
DHS conflict content: Conflict of not wanting to smell

Explanation: If the loss of the sense of smell is not just temporary but permanent, we are dealing with a track that developed during a conflict of "being unable to stand the smell".

An animal avoids the smell it has experienced once as being unbearable.

But since we humans "force" ourselves through the tracks again and again, the body helps itself and the nose "shuts down".

Example:
CA phase: Loss of sense of smell

PCL phase:
The sense of smell is coming back after the healing phase is completed; epileptic crisis is not critical even if the conflict lasts a long time, or the tracks are permanent.

Shoulder pain
DHS conflict content: SWE in the mother/child relationship or relationship between partners

Handedness: E.g., left-handed woman: Right shoulder – mother/child conflict; right-handed woman: Right shoulder – partner conflict

Example:
"I am a bad mother/bad daughter" or "I am a bad partner"

CA phase: Bone osteolyses in this area

PCL phase: Edema and expansion of the periosteum, pain, recalcification, leukemia, and joint rheumatism (in the traditional medicine often diagnosed as arthritis)

The recalcification corresponds with the diagnosis of the traditional medicine: Osteosarcoma

Germ layer: Mesoderm

A partner is everyone except a person's own mother or a person's own child.

See also: SWE

Sinusitis
See: Head cold

Skullcap pain
(Calotte pain)

DHS conflict content: SWE in the intellectual area (injustice, feeling of being bound, strife, etc.)

Example:
A person is accused of being incompetent in his or her own field.

CA phase: Bone osteolyses in this area

PCL phase: Edema and expansion of the periosteum, pain, recalcification, and leukemia

Germ layer: Mesoderm
See also: SWE

SM
SM = traditional medicine

Soft tissue rheumatism
DHS conflict content:

A) separation conflict and hurting someone else, or

B) separation conflict and suffering from periosteum pain oneself

Example:
Hurting someone else (mentally or mechanically) or: Someone hurt me. If the feeling of "being hurt" results in a separation conflict, so-called rheumatism develops. In most cases it is linked to a SWE.

173

A teenager wants to meet with friends and knows only roughly where the meeting point is. In addition, he is late. Because of the hurry, and because he is keeping an eye out for his friends, instead of watching what happens in front of him, he runs into a lamp post (= painful bump on the head) and doesn't find his friends at all (separation conflict).

Consequence: Paresthesia in the affected area for about a year

CA phase: Numbness in the affected area where the pain was inflicted or experienced. The bone healing edema (of the injury inflicted by oneself!) as well as pain can result in a local sensory paralysis.

PCL phase: Severe, "flowing pain" (rheumatism), minor swelling

Germ layer: Ectoderm

Solitary liver carcinoma
Biological conflict content: Starvation conflict, existence conflict

Example:
Extreme (unexpected) lack of money, but also fear of starving due to colorectal cancer

CA phase: Typical round so-called "solitary nodules, which appear dark in the CAT scan. Often, colorectal carcinoma, liver carcinoma, and pancreas carcinoma occur simultaneously during the same "overlapping conflict".

PCL phase: The healing can come about in different ways.
1. Encapsulation (the liver can add new tissue for the lost liver parenchyma)
2. Caseating decomposition, e.g., through TB: Liver TB. One kind of liver cirrhosis is the form of liver TB the connective tissue of which is healed up and which has compressed liver caverns. The other kind is described under intrahepatic bile duct ulcer and hepatitis, respectively.

Germ layer: Endoderm

Hamer Focus in the brain: HH in the right lateral pons

Sources
Sources used for this glossary:

- different books and other publications by Dr. Ryke Geerd Hamer

- content of the website www.pilhar.com

- personal statements of the therapist Daniela Amstutz

- personal statements of other affected people, e.g., contributions to the different forums as well as entries taken from the encyclopedia of the GNM forum www.gnm-forum.ws

- encyclopedia from lexikon.freenet.de

- medical technical literature

"Speech tinnitus"
Tinnitus triggered by words instead of noises

See:
Tinnitus
Acute hearing loss
Schizophrenia in terms of the traditional medicine

Hearing voices
Paranoia

Stomach cancer
DHS conflict content: Conflict of "having swallowed the chunk already but being unable to digest it".
Indigestible conflict

Example:
A good deal doesn't come through; a lawsuit is lost

CA phase: Cauliflower-like growing stomach carcinoma

PCL phase: Tumor decomposition through fungi or mycobacteria. If not already encapsulated, encapsulation takes place.

Germ layer: Endoderm
See also differentiation toward:
Stomach ulcer

Stomach pain
See: Stomach ulcer

Stomach ulcer
Duodenal ulcer (bulbus duodeni)
Gastritis
"Stomach pain"

DHS conflict content: Territory trouble

Handedness:
Right-handed woman:
Conflict 1 – identity conflict (rectum carcinoma), conflict 2 – (as female side of the brain already blocked, now experienced in a male fashion, e.g.:) – territory trouble (stomach ulcer)

Left-handed woman:
Conflict 1 - identity conflict (stomach ulcer), conflict 2 - (as male side of the brain already blocked, experienced in a female fashion again, e.g.:) – another identity conflict (rectum carcinoma)

Right-handed man:
Conflict 1 – territory trouble (stomach ulcer), conflict 2 - (as male side of the brain blocked, now experienced in a female fashion, e.g.:) - identity conflict (rectum carcinoma)

Left-handed man:
Conflict 1 - Conflict 1 – territory quarrels (rectum carcinoma), (as female side of the brain blocked, experienced in a male fashion again, e.g.:) – another conflict of territory quarrels (stomach ulcer)

Example:
A co-worker takes it for granted to spread his files all over the colleague's filing space, so that the colleague ends up lacking space for his or her own files.

Wife cheats on her husband; car gets a dent.

In general: Someone or something intrudes somebody else's territory (territory quarrels)

Not knowing which direction to turn to, or which opinion to agree with (identity conflict)

CA phase: Ulcer development (stomach)

PCL phase: Bleeding of the ulcers, gastritis (stomach)

Germ layer: Ectoderm
See:
Rectum carcinoma
Hemorrhoids

See also differentiation toward:
Stomach cancer

Stress urinary incontinence
Conflict of territory marking

See also: Occlusion of the urethra

Stroke
White/red

This topic is by far too complex for an exact description within the limits of this encyclopedia. See for this Dr. Hamer's original tables. The following outline can't be more than a first introduction.

DHS conflict content:
Conflict content of the face palsy: Losing one's face, having made a fool of oneself.

Conflict content of the palsy of the extremities: Unable to detect danger, followed by the conflict of being left alone, conflict of losing contact with one's family.

Example:
Sensory conflict -
A person pretends with his or her family to be someone or to have something he or she is not or has not. The family finds out about it, which constitutes the "loss of face" for the person. At the same time, he or she realizes that there is the risk of the fraud becoming known, but he or she can't tell where the danger is coming from. When the fraud actually does become known, the family turns away from the person, or he or she turns away out of shame, etc. (conflict: Unable to detect danger, after that: Being left, breaking tie on the family's part).

CA phase: Palsy, so-called white stroke

PCL phase: Resolution of palsy symptoms

Seizure during a sensory conflict: Absence

Germ layer: Ectoderm

Addendum: It is differentiated between a white (ischemic) and a red (hemorrhagic) stroke. A white stroke shows the palsies of the CA phase (see above). Often, during a red stroke, a severely edematized and already porous HH bursts and palsies occur in the PCL phase – mostly because a conflict lasted too long, was too intense, or there are repeated relapses (see also: Multiple sclerosis). That can be every conflict in the healing phase.

In case of speech loss: The affected artery is the one leading through Broca's area (motor cortex), or a relay impairing Broca's area, respectively, and, thus, results in speech loss.

See also:
Parkinson's
Multiple sclerosis

Struma
See: Thyroid dysfunctions

Stuttering
See speech loss under keyword: Stroke

Sudden Cardiac Death (SCD)
DHS conflict content: SWF in physical performance, "I don't want to do this any longer, I can't do it any more; how can I manage all of this?"

Example:
"Unexplainable" sudden cardiac death of an athlete in the middle of his training

CA phase: The heart muscle itself is affected.

PCL phase: Heart attack in the epileptic crisis (myocardial infarction [AMI or MI]; the heart muscle can tear in the process), if the conflict has been lasting for a very long time, or the person doesn't listen to his or her body and keeps putting strain on it. Consequently, it is impossible for the heart muscle to relax.

See also the differentiation: Heart attack

Support association
www.faktor-L.de

SWE
SWE = collapse of self-esteem; a conflict content

See also under:
Hand joint pain
Foot joint pain
Knee pain
Shoulder pain
Neck pain
Pubic bone pain
Skullcap pain
Back pain
Hip joint pain
Polyarthritis
Gout

Myoma
Varicose veins
Lupus
Stroke

Swelling of the nasal mucosa
See: Head cold

Syndrome
The condition of extreme accumulation of excess fluid in the body is called syndrome.

In order to bring about a syndrome, two criteria have to be fulfilled:

First criterion:

There has to be an active conflict (conflict active phase, CA phase), the associated SBS of which includes the accumulation of excess fluid (kidney tubular water retention; the body conserves water, because it may not find water fast enough in an unknown environment). This is the case with conflict contents that are based on the feeling of being lost, e.g., a refugee conflict.

Second criterion:

There has to be another conflict that has been resolved (conflict resolved- or healing phase = PCL- or CL phase).

Consequence:

The fluid accumulation of the active conflict is enormously reinforced by the edema formation during the healing phase. This condition continues up to the epileptoid crisis. Special attention has to be paid here to the edema (Hamer Focus [HH]) in the brain. Due to the massive accumulation of fluid, the brain pressure can increase and reach an extremely high and life-threatening value.

This is one of the reasons why it is strongly recommended that people don't start working on their conflicts without an experienced therapist, especially if someone suffers from an active refugee conflict.

Note:
A possible home remedy for the symptoms is taking baths in a saline solution, the efficiency of which has different reasons. One of them is the fact that salts withdraw water from the body (osmosis).

176

Recipe for the bath:
Take 3 tbsp of Jentschura and Lohkämper Orgon salt and let it dissolve in the bathtub at body temperature; duration of the bath: 1/2 – 2 hours. You can also use 1 kg rock salt dissolved in the tub. Sea salt possibly serves a similar purpose.

The baths are also supposed to reduce the conflict mass of each conflict. Full baths should only be taken after consultation with a therapist, as they may not be indicated for people with heart problems.

Thrush
See: Aphthous oral infection

Thyroid dysfunctions
Hyperthyreosis, Basedow's disease, hypothyreosis, myxedema

DHS conflict content: Hyperthyreosis
A) being unable to get rid of (transporting) something into the intestine due to lacking hormone secretion;

B) unable to grasp a desired chunk (food) – because the individual isn't fast enough

Example:
A) not having sold off idle shares at the right time

B) a sales person's colleague snaps up the customers because she is faster, so that the sales person barely has any sales herself

CA phase: Tumor growth, "hard struma" with hyperthyreosis (increased thyroxine production)

PCL phase: Tumor decomposition through TB bacteria, after that thyroxine production returns to normal. If TB bacteria are not already existent at the time the DHS occurs, the tumor encapsulates and the thyroxine production doesn't return to normal, resulting in hyperthyreosis despite a conflict resolution.

DHS conflict content: Hypothyreosis - Conflict of being powerless: "My hands are tied, I can't do anything", or "Somebody should really do something, but nobody does anything".

Example:
An individual feels helpless and powerless in regards to politics, which are perceived as unfair (conflict content vulnerable to relapses)

CA phase: Cystic obstruction of the thyroid ducts, ulcer in the thyroid ducts (in order to produce more thyroxine), not visible, possibly sometimes dragging pain in the thyroid.

PCL phase: Thyroid cysts (euthyroid), struma (benign goiter), cold nodules, normalization of the hormone production, or hypothyreosis (decreased thyroxine production).

See also:
Hypothyreosis
Myxedema
Hyperthyreosis
Basedow's disease
Struma
Goiter
Cold nodules

Tinnitus
DHS conflict content: Hearing conflict, conflict of "not wanting to hear", "Did I hear right?" "I can't believe what I am hearing!"

CA phase: Tinnitus in the ear (whistling, humming, ringing, roaring), increasing hearing loss

PCL phase: Acute hearing loss, edema in the inner ear

Germ layer: Ectoderm

Characteristic: Tinnitus can occur in both ears. This corresponds with a second hearing conflict affecting the other ear, which puts the patient into schizophrenic constellation. If it is "speech tinnitus", patients hear voices; otherwise they hear unbearable noises in both ears.

See also:
Hearing voices
Schizophrenia

Tonsils, craggy
See: Inflammation of the tonsils

Tonsil hyperplasia
See: Inflammation of the tonsils

Tonsil hypertrophy
See: Inflammation of the tonsils

Tonsillitis
See: Inflammation of the tonsils

Track
See: Tracks

Tracks
In the moment of the DHS, a person registers the circumstances during the experience and possibly associates them with the experience as such. This can be a sensory stimulus, for example, a smell, etc., which, after the resolution of the initial conflict, leads to a new relapse (repetition of the Meaningful Special Biological Program) every time the person is exposed to that particular circumstance, although he or she doesn't suffer another DHS. The person hit a so-called track. That's how allergies work as well.

See also:
SBS
DHS
Allergy

Trigeminal neuralgia
Occurs in relapses of separation conflicts (e.g., neurodermatitis episodes), breaking ties with the family, no physical contact

See: Neurodermatitis

Tumor mycosis
Caseating, necrotizising decomposition of a tumor through fungi

Ulcers
Ulcers are "holes" in the tissue. They develop (according to the New Medicine) during the CA phase after a SBS in the cerebral cortex.

Examples are:
- Osteolysis (porous bones or bone loss),
- Lung nodules,
- Decomposition of arteries, and
- Decomposition of the inner walls of the coronary vessels.

In both examples, tissue is decomposed during the conflict active phase. In the PCL phase, however, these holes are filled again, resulting in:

- Stronger bones (in case of a previous osteolysis), the strengthening of which is occasionally called "bone cancer" by the traditional medicine,

- Cicatrisation in the lung tissue

- Calcified arteries and coronary vessels

Valvular heart disease
See: Endocarditis

Varices
See: Varicose veins

Varicose veins
(Varices)
Phlebitis
DHS conflict content: SWE, leg veins = "ball and chain" conflict

Example:
After the birth of her child, the mother has to care for it all the time; she perceives it as a "ball and chain" (leg varices).

CA phase: Vein spasms, varicose veins; visible with several conflict relapses (blood vessel necroses)

PCL phase: Expanding, swelling veins, so-called varices. Phlebitis (= healing of the damaged wall of the vein)

Germ layer: Mesoderm

Waterhouse-Friedrichsen syndrome
See: Cushing's syndrome

White stroke
See: Stroke

Status: October 2005

Epilogue

"Do you know what I think is absolutely cool about the New Medicine?" My son, Philipp, asked me this question while we were on a comfortable long endurance run. The pace was such that we could talk without problems and, as always, the distance was in accordance with to the topics of our conversation. After this introduction, however, it was clear to me that this run would take at least 90 minutes. "So? What is the cool thing?" I asked as was expected of me, and he responded, "That it takes away the fear."

At this point, Philipp obviously put a big period behind his thought. He was silent for about three seconds. Before I could agree with him he continued, "In the past, I was afraid of viruses, bacteria, this and that disease, strange knobs and lumps, pain, and what not. Today, if I detect something, I start looking for the reason why it would develop. And I know it is nothing serious. Even if it hurts, even if it takes a long time, or I don't find the cause right away, I am not afraid any more."

At this moment, I started to realize that Hamer's discovery was more than simply a New Medicine. (To be correct, it should just be called Medicine. If one really wants to make distinctions, surely it would be more appropriate to rename the currently practiced medicine, which is regarded as the standard, Old Medicine.) It is a relief. If you know about it, understand its connections, and can use it, you are free of fear and free for other things. Without fear, people can live their lives; if they are fearful, they can exist at best.

This realization isn't really new. But to know it and to feel it are two different things. This fall, I was able to directly experience once again how fear had a grip on many people. This time, the alleged danger was called bird flu. About 60 people worldwide have allegedly died of the virus, which hasn't been proven yet.

Because of that fear, millions of birds lost their lives. In Romania, they were buried alive, strangled, or slain. People carried out a downright massacre—out of fear. In Germany, frightened people called authorities and demanded for all migratory birds to be shot, because they would present too much of a danger. Chicken farmers have to lock up their animals in dark stables, where some of them will certainly go stir-crazy.

The fear has deprived our neighborhood of an attraction as well. In the middle of the city next to a nursery there is a big enclosed meadow. Until recently, chickens of all breeds scratched for worms and bugs in this meadow. Parents with small children weren't the only ones using it as a destination. The parents spoiled the chicken with breadcrumbs and the kids imitated the clucking.

The male nurses of the adjacent retirement home rolled the wheel chairs with the old men and women to this place as well. The old people livened up here, laughed, and talked to the animals; some of them tried to crow. They were as happy as the little children. And every morning, I enjoyed hearing the crowing of the rooster. It was an adventure people could have in the middle of the city—until fear came. It deprived families of their destination, the old people of a pleasure of life, me of the pleasant memory in the morning, and the chickens of the sun, the wind, and their freedom.

Since I stopped smoking three years ago – not for alleged health reasons, but because I noticed that smoking makes me dependent (Honestly, as a smoker you can't even treat yourself to a trip through the desert. How can you explain that you can't take that much water because you have to leave space for several cartons of cigarettes?) – my nose has become even more sensitive and, sometimes, the smell of tobacco is bothering me.

But when I see the scaremongering that is supposed to take away every little bit of fun from smokers, when I see how millions of Euros are invested in anti-smoking campaigns and drugs that are supposed to help smokers give up smoking instead of letting people have their personal freedom, I feel occasionally inclined to give some smoker, who is standing around with a guilty look on their face, a tap on the shoulder and light them a cigarette.

Fear has a long history. Some few people have always used it to their advantage. In the 16th century, for example, the monk, Johann Tetzel as one of many others sold indulgences. He himself was afraid of hell and believed firmly in their effectiveness. The beneficiary was Pope Leo, who used the money to finance his plans. Considering this, it becomes perfectly clear how important Martin Luther really was for the world. He was a liberator. By translating the bible and, thus, making it also available to the people without education, he took away their fear and, at the same time, the pope's tool. Knowledge was the key here as well.

You don't have to go back in history too far in order to find such examples. During this fall, the bird flu is such an example. For the coming years, the World Bank anticipates expenditures as high as three billion Euros to fight the bird flu, the costs for drugs not included. Shortly before the election, the people in charge at the german Robert Koch Institute didn't stop beating a path to the door of the outgoing finance minister, Hans Eichel until he allowed 20 million Euros for vaccination research.

Last year, SARS was the worldwide fear monger. Today, this alleged lung disease isn't worth another line any longer. Several years earlier, BSE was the culprit; also not to be forgotten is the fear of anthrax terror attacks.

Or let's take the fear of Jews, which can be found throughout the centuries. Many people used that fear to pocket the possessions of their Jewish fellow citizens, and Hitler exploited it to eventually lead an annihilation campaign against the Jews unequalled to this day. Again, fear was the willing helper of the perpetrators.

US President George Bush stoked fears of a strong Iraq allegedly building nuclear weapons or other weapons of mass destruction. And when the American people were so frightened they would have agreed to anything, he marched in.

They didn't find weapons of mass destruction, which they apologized for with a lame "Sorry". Meanwhile, the war in Iraq has developed into a civil war, as every observer halfway blessed with common sense had predicted. But, at least, the United States got a little closer to the oil resources.

People who are not afraid can't be manipulated. They are truly free. Hamer's New Medicine is an important factor for this personal freedom for everybody. The german virologist, Dr. Stefan Lanka, who persistently challenges and researches, is another one. And a third one is Frank Stelzer and the Stelzer engine, which won't be built, because it would mean too much freedom.

However, all these discoveries or inventions wouldn't mean anything without the people who understood them and, thus, see to it that they become accepted. The fact that it hasn't happened yet in the three cases mentioned and in several others either shows that there are not enough of these people around yet.

The purpose of this book is to help increase the number of these people. It wants to take your fear away. It is an offer. Read, understand, and, above all—live!

Monika Berger-Lenz – October 2005

A Final Word
• Panic – and who benefits from it

It is not very often that the editor of a book has the chance to provide the reader with an instrument for the short-term check of a scientific prognosis or statement directed towards the future. This is one of these rare opportunities.

You can check the New Medicine right away for yourself and your environment if you use this handbook accordingly. But we would like to give you another possibility to get an idea of the so-called scientific statements and announcements.

The general panic concerning the commencing bird flu epidemic just reached its climax. Enormous amounts of money have been provided to develop or buy vaccines.

We (FAKTuell) did an interview with Dr. Stefan Lanka, in which he comes to a completely different conclusion than the politicians and the traditional medicine. Until the summer of 2006, you have the opportunity to observe and check whose statement is right.

If, after BSE and SARS, the bird flu, as well, was only "invented" as an instrument to unscrupulously earn money, that is, if Dr. Lanka is right, than it will be easier for you, dear readers, to concern yourselves or even reconcile with so-called outsider arguments in the future.

The question we as enlightened people always need to ask first when confronted with official announcements and statements, particularly those with such a huge panic potential, is this: Who is going to benefit?!

*Christopher Ray * October 2005*

No Panic –
The Truth about Bird Flu, H5N1, Vaccines, and AIDS
Christopher Ray * Commentary and Interview October 10, 2005

If you watch the meddling with symptoms and how it is practiced during the current coalition negotiations, you can't take the announcements of the politicians and their gofers seriously any more.
Or do you really believe that even one single job will be created by further cutting Hartz IV and ALG II (unemployment insurance and social assistance)?
Or that the big job wave will inevitably happen if we cut taxes for companies, increase contributions to health insurance and value-added tax, and cut or abolish the commuter flat rate and the night shift premiums? All this despite daily news about jobs being cut and companies being closed down...

If you swallow all this without contradiction, you may as well do the same with the spoonful of sugar that will help to get your next vaccine down and delete this page from your website favourites in favour of those whose titles and headlines are written in capital letters.
However, if you are aware that you are constantly being taken for a fool and are being downright kidded (excuse the language!), then you should take some time and listen to an independent scientist who has not been bought yet: Virologist Dr. rer.nat. Stefan Lanka.
He answered all the questions the FAKTuell editorial department asked him– without any backdoors.

Here is the interview:

Bird Flu and H5N1, Vaccinating, and AIDS

Dr. Lanka, are we in Germany threatened by the bird flu?

Only indirectly. Next year we will have a lot less babies in Germany. If you follow the media, all the storks will be carried off by the bird flu. We should prepare ourselves for that.

Are you serious?

As serious as I am about any other imminent danger for us from the alleged bird flu virus H5N1. The danger or the disaster lies somewhere else entirely.

In your opinion, where lies the danger or the disaster?

We were broken of the habit of using our brains. That is the actual danger or the catastrophe. Politicians and the media take it upon themselves to delude us into believing everything, for example, delude us into thinking that migratory birds in Asia have been infected with a very dangerous, deadly virus. These fatally ill birds then keep flying for weeks on end.

They fly for thousands of kilometers, infect chickens, geese, and other poultry in Rumania, Turkey, Greece, etc., with which they didn't have contact, but which get sick and die within a very short time. However, the migratory birds don't get sick and die, but keep flying for weeks, thousands of kilometers. If you believe that, you also believe that the stork brings the babies. In fact, the majority of people in Germany do believe in a bird flu threat.

184

So, *does the bird flu exist at all?*

Diseases in poultry from intensive mass animal farming have been found since the late 19th century: blue coloration of the crown, decrease of the egg production, dull coat, and sometimes the animals die. These diseases were called bird pest.

In today's mass poultry farming, particularly when chickens are kept in cages, many animals die on a daily basis as a consequence of animal farming foreign to the species. Later, these consequences of intensive mass animal farming were no longer called bird pest, but bird flu. For decades, we have been told that these diseases are caused by a transferable virus in order to distract from the real causes.

Those 100 million *chickens that apparently died of the bird flu actually died in reality of stress and/or deficiency and poisoning?*

No! If a chicken lays fewer eggs, or its crown turns blue, and it also tests positive for H5N1, all other chickens are being gased. That's how those 100 million chickens came about that were apparently killed by the H5N1 virus.

If you have a closer look, you can detect the strategy behind this process, which has been used for decades. In the West, big farms are being compensated for the animals that died of the "pest." They will be refunded at the highest market price at the expense of the general public, while the poultry market in Asia and everywhere else where poultry is farmed successfully is willfully and deliberately destroyed under the instruction of the UN organization FAO (United Nation's Food and Agriculture Organization).
That's why all big Western poultry farmers keep their mouths shut and, through their veterinarians, make sure that, if the market price for poultry decreases, they get the diagnosis of an infectious disease which allows them to "dispose" of their animals - in fact all at the same time - with a greater gain than would be possible through normal farming at the state-guaranteed maximum price.

To reduce it to a common denominator: It is modern economic subsidy fraud combined with producing paralyzing fear, guaranteeing that nobody is asking for proof along the way.

What was the cause of death of the 61 people *who proved to have the H5N1 virus?*

There are only very few reports accessible for the public, describing the shown symptoms and how these symptoms were treated. These cases are clear: People with cold symptoms who had the misfortune to fall into the hands of H5N1-hunters were killed with enormously high doses of chemotherapy supposed to slow down the phantom virus. Isolated in plastic tents and surrounded by lunatics in space suits, they died angst-ridden of multiple organ failure.

Are you saying then that this bird flu virus *doesn't actually exist?*

Structures that could be referred to as bird flu viruses, or influenza viruses, or any other virus said to cause disease have never been detected or seen in humans, in blood or other body fluids, in animals, or in a plant.

The causes of diseases, even those in animals, that are said to have been caused by a virus, and which occur fast, successively, or simultaneously in several individuals, have been known for a long time. Even more: There is simply no biological evidence for viruses as the cause of a disease.

Only if you persistently ignore the findings of Dr. Hamer's New Medicine, saying that traumatic events are the cause of many diseases, as well as the findings in chemistry about the effects of poisoning and deficiencies, and the findings in physics about the effects of radiation, then there's room for woolgathering like viruses that make you sick.

Then why do *people still insist on viruses as the cause of a disease?*

Traditional physicians need the paralyzing, stupefying, and destructive fear of phantom viruses that cause diseases as the pivotal basis of their existence: firstly, to harm large numbers of people by vaccinating them and, thus, to create a clientele of chronically ill and ailing objects who won't object to anything that is being done to them.

Secondly, to not have to admit to themselves that they fail completely in treating chronic diseases, and that they killed and are still killing more people than all the wars did so far. Every traditional physician is aware of this, but only very few dare to speak about it. Therefore, it is not surprising that the suicide rate in traditional physicians is by far the highest compared to other occupation groups.

Thirdly, traditional physicians need the paralyzing, stupefying, and destructive fear of devilish viruses to cover up their origin as the instrument of oppression and killing of the aspiring Vatican, which, in turn, developed from the insurgent West-Roman army.

Traditional medicine has been and still is the most important foothold of all dictatorships and governments that don't want to comply with written law, the constitutions, human rights, that is, to the democratically legitimized social contract. This also explains why the traditional medicine can and is allowed to do virtually everything it pleases, and is subject to no control at all. If we don't overcome this situation, we will all die by this traditional medicine.

Aren't you exaggerating *a little?*

Unfortunately, no! Everyone who opens his or her eyes will come to see it this way.

Ivan Illich already warned against it in his 1975 analysis *Die Enteignung der Gesundheit* (*The Expropriation of Health*). This book is still available today under the title *Die Nemesis der Medizin* (*Medical Nemesis*).

Goethe very accurately described the state of the traditional medicine in *Faust I* when he has Dr. Faustus admit:

186

Here was the medicine, the patients died and nobody asked who convalesced, so we ravaged with hellish electuaries worse than the pestilence in these valleys, these mountains; I myself administered the poison to thousands; they withered, I had to witness that the brazen murderers were praised.

Goethe calls the traditional physicians who administer the electuaries, that is, the poisonous substances, brazen murderers, who even today are being praised. Here, I can and I also must refer to our publications, because we were the first to ask the modern medicine the crucial question and documented and commented the confessions. At www.klein-klein-aktion.de and www.klein-klein-verlag.de you can find all the relevant information.

How did you of all people stumble on this millennium fraud?

I studied molecular biology.

During my studies I found the first virus in the sea in sea algae. This evidence of a virus was first published in 1990 in a scientific publication in accordance with the standard of natural sciences. The virus I found propagates inside the sea algae, it can leave it, and it can propagate again in other algae of this kind without having any negative effect, and this virus is not connected to any disease.

For instance, in one liter of seawater you have over 100 million different viruses. Fortunately, the health authorities and the doctors aren't aware of this yet, otherwise there would long be a law that allows swimming in the sea only in a full body condom.

Biological structures, however, that would have negative effects have never been found. The basis of biological life is cooperation, is symbiosis, and there is no room for war and destruction. Only sick and criminal minds accredit war and destruction to biological life.

During my studies, I as well as other people have not been able to find any evidence for the existence of disease-causing viruses. Later, we reported these results publicly and invited people to not take our word for it either, but to check for themselves whether disease-causing viruses exist.

From this, the klein-klein campaign developed, which, for over 5 years, has been asking health authorities for evidence and, in the end, received the admission and the certainty that there is no evidence for disease-causing viruses, and no evidence for the benefit of vaccinating either. Three years ago, we founded the klein-klein verlag in order to be able to publish these results unaltered.

Which viruses actually exist and what effect do they have?

Structures that can be called viruses exist in many kinds of bacteria and in simple life forms that are still similar to bacteria. They are elements of different cells living together in a common cell type, which have remained independent. That is called a symbiosis, an endosymbiosis, resulting from the process of merging of different cell types and structures the current cell type emanated from and humans, animals, and plants consist of.

187

Like the mitochondria, the bacteria in all our cells, which breathe our oxygen, or the chloroplasts, the bacteria in all plants, which produce oxygen, viruses are components of cells.

Very important: Viruses are components of very simple organisms like, for instance, string algae, a certain kind of single-celled chlorella algae, and a great number of bacteria. In bacteria, these viral components are called phages. In more complex organisms like humans in particular, or animals and plants, however, such structures that could be called viruses have never been found.

Contrary to the mitochondria, bacteria in our cells, or the chloroplasts, the bacteria in every plant, that are unable to leave the common cell, because they are dependent on the common cell's metabolism, viruses can leave the cells, since they don't have any function within the cell crucial for the survival.

So, viruses are cell components that have given their entire metabolism to the common cell and, therefore, can leave the cell. Outside the common cell, they help other cells by transferring construction- and energy substances. No other function has ever been observed.

The actual scientifically proven viruses have a helping and supporting function instead of a destroying one within the highly complex processes among the cells.

Also, when we look at diseases, no structure has ever been found or isolated in a sick organism or in body fluids that could be called a virus. It is a transparent fraud and a fatal lie with dramatic consequences to claim that there exists some kind of disease-causing virus.

You don't suggest that the dangerous AIDS virus is only a virtual virus as well, do you?

It is not only I who is suggesting that the so-called AIDS virus "HIV" has never been scientifically proven, but is only considered proven as a result of a consensus. On January 5, 2004, the federal minister of health, Ulla Schmidt, wrote to the member of the Bundestag, Rudolf Kraus, "Of course, in the international scientific consensus the Human Immunodeficiency Virus is considered scientifically proven."

Today, after citizens have been asking the federal health authorities repeatedly year after year for scientific proof regarding the suggested disease-causing viruses, the federal health authorities no longer maintain that some virus claimed to be a pathogen was directly proven. In an ongoing petition process before the German Bundestag, the Federal Ministry of Health passed the responsibility on to the Federal Ministry of Research. The Federal Ministry of Research is now of the absurd opinion, that the freedom of the sciences as protected in the Basic Constitutional Law forbids the state to check the assertions of the sciences.

That is just absurd. It would mean that the state is handing us over to an uncontrolled science that can do whatever it pleases without any protection for us. Do you really think that the state is handing us over in such a way?

188

I don't have an opinion here. I can just point to the facts. We are experiencing in the current bird flu panic how the government in Germany against better judgment hands the population over to some people who camouflage themselves as scientists. An enforced chemotherapy is planned, and in the spring the entire German population is to be forcibly vaccinated twice against the suggested bird flu phantom.

But neither has a bird flu virus ever been detected nor has any virus been detected that was connected in any way to a disease. Such viruses don't exist. They are being considered proven, and, thus, claimed existent the same way the minister admitted in regards to the suggested AIDS virus: based on an international scientific consensus.

But the bird flu virus H5N1, which is dangerous to humans, *has been clearly identified in an English laboratory during the last days.*

If ever a virus was found in a concrete body or a fluid, for instance in birds, every mediocre scientist in a mediocre laboratory can check within a day whether this virus is existent in a dead animal. But this never happened. On the contrary, the people responsible use indirect and completely irrelevant test methods that tell absolutely nothing.

For example, some people claim that there are antibodies that exclusively attach to the body of the suggested virus, so when there is evidence of a reaction between body and antibody the existence of the virus is proven. In reality, the suggested antibodies are soluble blood proteins, which play a pivotal role in the sealing of growing and dividing cells and in wound healing. These blood proteins, also called globulins, in the test tube bind arbitrarily to other proteins if they find appropriate concentrations of acids and bases, minerals, and solvents. Thus, you can test any sample of an animal or a human positive or negative. It has to be said quite clearly that this is a matter of purely criminal arbitrariness.

Some people claim that, by using a biochemical amplification technique called polymerase chain reaction (PCR), the so-called genetic material of the virus was multiplied and, thus, proven to exist, but that is fraud. First, there is no genetic material of a disease-causing virus, with which the artificially amplified particles can be compared and, second, only those particles of the genetic material are multiplied that were already in the fluids used to indirectly prove the suggested virus.

And yet it is so easy:

A thousand pieces of indirect evidence like, for instance, crop circles don't make an UFO either. You don't even have to know English in order to read the publications the virus frauds are referring to, and to find out for yourself that there isn't a virus mentioned anywhere. If you ask these scientists for the evidence that proves the existence of the alleged viruses, for example, the H5N1 virus, you will only get excuses but never a concrete answer.

On TV, we have heard over and over again that the tests were carried out in an English laboratory. The public has never learned the name of this English laboratory. It is the EU's reference laboratory for bird flu in Weybridge. I have asked the scientists several times for evidence regarding the existence of the

H5N1 virus. They replied just once and then never again; they wrote that they didn't understand my question.

I also wrote several times to the World Health Organization and in particular to the coordinator of the bird flu pandemic, the German, Klaus Stöhr, to ask for evidence concerning the existence of the bird flu virus. Neither the WHO nor Klaus Stöhr responded.

But what exactly means H5N1, *which the whole world is afraid of?*

The "H" in H5N1 stands for hemagglutinin, the "N" stands for neuraminidase. The pseudo-virologists claim that the shells of the flu viruses contain proteins of the type hemagglutinin and proteins of the enzyme neuramidase.

In biochemistry, many different substances besides proteins agglutinating red blood cells are called hemagglutinin.

The pseudo-virologists agreed that the shells of flu viruses should contain 15 different kinds of proteins with the characteristics of a hemagglutinin. The "5" stands for type five of a suggested protein, which, again, can only be proven indirectly. So, in order to prove a flu virus, red blood cell are mixed with samples that supposedly contain the alleged virus. If the red blood cells agglutinate, these virologists claim that the cause for the agglutination must be a hemagglutinin in a flu virus, although they have never isolated a virus from this sample or such a mixture, let alone having seen one.

From the way the agglutination occurred they then conclude, like the seers in the cartoon *Asterix and Obelix*, which type of hemagglutinin has been found. These scientists have a multitude of testing procedures at their disposal, ensuring through their set up that they indicate exactly the type of hemagglutinin the "testing" scientist had already assumed beforehand.

The same applies to the enzyme neuramidase, which is claimed to be a component of the shells of flu viruses. The pseudo-virologists claim 9 different types of this enzyme. In reality, the neuramidase is one enzyme, which, by separating parts of an amino sugar called neuramin acid, regulates the surface tension, which is crucial for the functioning of the respective metabolism. Analogous to the "viral" hemagglutinin, there are multitudinous corrupt testing procedures that "show" exactly the result, that is, the particular type of neuramidase the "seeing" virologist had already assumed beforehand.

Consequently, it is no surprise that the turkey belonging to the 73-year-old farmer Dimitris Kominaris from the East Aegaen island of Inousses, which apparently died of H5N1, disappeared without a trace; or that a sample from Greece demonstrably never arrived at the reference laboratory in question, but the clear-sighted media reported that a first sample confirmed the suspicion. In order to provide evidence for H5N1, no sample is necessary, indeed, because it is a matter of a planned action to create fear for political reasons, as is the case with all alleged epidemics.

The media are constantly showing photos of bird flu- and influenza viruses. Some of these photos show round structures. Aren't those viruses?

No! First of all, the round structures that are supposed to be flu viruses are artificially produced particles consisting of fats and proteins, as is obvious for any molecular biologist.

The layman can check this by asking for a scientific publication that shows these pictures, describes them, and documents the composition of these particles. Such a publication doesn't exist.

Secondly, it is clearly evident for every biologist that these pictures, which supposedly show bird flu viruses, are images of completely normal cell components, or even entire cells in the process of exporting or importing cell- and metabolism components. Again, the layman can easily check this by asking for the underlying publications the pictures were taken from. He or she will never receive such publications. The scare mongers' guild doesn't like to reveal the basis of its business, which is the fraud concerning laboratory- and animal testing.

If you ask the photo agencies and dpa (German Press Agency) where they get their photos, they refer to the American epidemic authority, Centers for Disease Control and Prevention (CDC), of the Pentagon. And that's exactly where the only photo of the alleged H5N1 comes from. This photo shows the longitudinal- and at the same time the cross-section of tubes in cells, which are caused to die in the test tube. In technical terminology, these little tubes are called microtubules; they serve as a means of transport and communication within the cell and during cell division.

But there is evidence that H5N1 kills chicken embryos and can be cultivated in eggs. Where's the rub?

These experiments have been used for over 100 years to "prove" the existence of quite different "viruses", for instance, also the suggested poxvirus. In these experiments, extracts are injected through the eggshell into the embryo. Depending on how much and where in the embryo the apparently "virus-infected" extract was injected, the embryo dies more or less quickly. It would also die, if the extracts were sterilized first.

These virologists consider this killing direct evidence for the existence of the respective virus as well as for the possibility to propagate the virus, and, at the same time, they pass it off as evidence for the isolation of the virus. From chicken embryos killed this way – millions of them die quietly at the vaccine producers each year - miscellaneous vaccines are being produced.

Besides chicken embryos, cells are also killed in test tubes to pass off the dying of these cells as evidence for the existence, the propagation, and the isolation of a disease-causing virus. But nowhere is a virus being isolated from a test tube, photographed in the electron microscope, and its components shown in procedures called electrophoresis.

But what if not H5N1 kills the animals in the animal experiments?

Again, you just have to have a look at the publications describing these experiments. Chickens are being slowly suffocated within three days by injecting fluid through the tube into their windpipe. Thirty days before the alleged infection, little Java monkeys get a temperature transmitter implanted in their abdomen; 5 days before the alleged infection they are fixated in a depression chamber, and when the so-called infection occurs, an amount of fluid corresponding to 8 jiggers for humans is pressed through the tube into the windpipes of these pups. Parts of the same extract from dying, that is, rotting, cells are injected into both eyes and the tonsils of the animals. Several times, the animals have to endure suffocation attacks, because their bronchi are flushed, and so on. The resulting damage and destruction is presented as the consequence of H5N1.

Through their personal consultants, I informed the former minister for consumer protection, Künast, and the current minister, Trittin, who pose as animal-rights activists, about this. There was no reaction.

But the Spanish flu virus *has been genetically reconstructed and it was determined that it is a bird flu virus!*

Only a model of the genetic material of an influenza virus was genetically reconstructed. A flu virus has never been isolated. A genetic substance of a flu virus has never been isolated either. All they did was to propagate genetic material via the biochemical propagating method of "Polymerase Chain Reaction". This method also allows propagating any number of new, short pieces of genetic material that never before existed.

This technique also allows manipulating the genetic fingerprint, that is, to test somebody identical to or different from a "found" sample. Provided it is performed properly, the genetic fingerprint gives a certain probability of a match, but only if you have a lot of genetic material to compare.

Dr. Jeffrey Taubenberger, who first claimed the reconstruction of the pandemic virus of 1918, is working for the US army and spent more than ten years producing short pieces of genetic material based on samples of different human bodies via the biochemical propagation technique PCR. From the multitude of produced pieces he chose those that came closest to the model of the genetic substance of the idea of a flu virus and he published them.

However, neither was a virus found or could be proven in any of the bodies, nor has a piece of genetic material been isolated from them. Out of nowhere, pieces of genetic material that weren't verifiable in the bodies before were created via the PCR technique. If viruses had existed, you would have been able to isolate them and their genetic material from them instead of tediously producing a rag rug of a genetic substance model of the idea of a flu virus via PCR with the clear intent to defraud.

How can the layman *check this?*

It is claimed that these short pieces, which are genetically incomplete and don't even meet the definition of a gene, if combined, would make the entire genetic material of a flu virus. In order to see through this fraud, you only have to be able to add the published lengths to conclude that the sum of the individual pieces' lengths, which are supposed to make the entire viral genetic material of the suggested flu virus, don't add up to the length of the idea of the flu virus model genome.

Easier, still, is it to ask in which publication you can find an electron-microscope photo of this apparently reconstructed virus. Such a publication doesn't exist.

It is claimed *that there were experiments showing that this reconstructed virus from 1918 would kill very effectively. What is wrong with this statement?*

If I inject a chicken embryo with a mixture of artificially produced pieces of genetic material and proteins directly into its heart, it will die faster than if I inject the mixture only peripherally.

If I expose cells in a test tube to a variety of artificially produced pieces of genetic material and proteins, they will die faster than under the standard conditions of cell death in the test tube, which are "normally" used to prove the existence, the isolation, and the propagation of the suggested viruses.

Based on this artificially produced genetic material that is passed off as viral, models of proteins are being created on the computer. Then, based on these protein models, the appearance of the entire virus is being reconstructed on the computer. That's all, but the world believes that it is possible to produce viruses in the lab. It also doesn't come as a surprise that, in reference to statements of the CIA and the British Secret Service, M16, it is claimed that the Communist regime in North Korea would now produce flu viruses even more deadly than H5N1.

Which conclusions *do you draw from that?*

Bin Laden, the leader of the suggested Al-Qaeda, which, in Arabic, just means "the path", hasn't been found and nobody has heard from this organization before the fire restoration of the collapse-endangered New Yorker skyscrapers. No weapons of mass destruction like the suggested poxviruses have been found in Saddam's Iraq, which were the reason for the second Iraq war. And now, deadly viruses are suggested once again. Considering these facts, it is pretty clear who are the real terrorists and who are the real suicide bombers: Everybody who participates in the virus panic and contributes to it!

In case the bird flu is proclaimed by the WHO, the pandemic plans include the possible breakdown of supplies and law and order. Estimates of up to 100 million dead people should be taken seriously.

I see a particular risk for all residents of retirement homes who, at the outbreak of chaos and the breakdown of the supply systems and law and order, will be the first and, besides small children, the unprotected and defenseless victims. It is scary to envision what would happen if the epidemic makers declared the state of emergency already during the winter.

How effective is the drug Tamiflu, *which is meanwhile being purchased with tax money and stored away, in protecting people from the bird flu?*

Nobody claims that this drug protects from the flu. Tamiflu is supposed to work as a neuramidase inhibitor. It inhibits the function of the sugar neuramin acid in the organism, which is, among others, responsible for the surface tension of the cells. The side effects of Tamiflu mentioned on the package insert are almost identical to the symptoms of a serious case of influenza.

So, drugs are now being stored in large quantities that cause exactly the same symptoms that occur in the case of a real, serious so-called flu. These symptoms will abate after seven days if you consult a doctor, and after a week if you don't.

If Tamiflu is given to sick people, it is likely to cause far more serious symptoms than those of a serious flu. If the pandemic in humans is declared, many people will take this drug at the same time, in which case we will actually have the clear symptoms of a Tamiflu epidemic. We will also have to expect people dying from Tamiflu, which, in turn, will be used as evidence for the dangerous nature of the bird flu and for the great care the state takes to protect people's health.

The well-tried AIDS pattern is being repeated. In Spain, it is written on the package insert that it is not known whether the symptoms are caused by the drugs or by the virus.

Then you won't recommend a general vaccination or the vaccination specifically developed for the bird flu?

I do not recommend insanity. Every vaccination contains toxins that have lasting effects, causing more or less severe permanent damage. The infection protection law requires the "**is**" as a necessary precondition for a vaccination being justified, that is, the existence of a pathogen, for example a virus.

Since none of the so-called disease-causing viruses can be or should be considered existent, there can also be no legal vaccination against the flu, and none against the bird flu either.

Every vaccination that has occurred in Germany after the infection protection law became effective on January 1, 2001, constitutes the felony of aggravated assault. Of course, I don't recommend for people to hand themselves over to become victims of felonies and crimes.

In your opinion, who is behind all of what we are currently experiencing here?

It can only be speculated. Naturally, the pharmaceutical industry is happy about the big business with the bird flu panic. But, actually, every single person is behind this insanity. The situation is what it is. It could only get to this point, because we as citizens allowed our state to act in such a way against the people, although, formally, our state is a democratic constitutional state.
If you wait for the pharmaceutical industry to change things for the good of the people, you will wait in vain. If you don't resist now, you don't live your life the right way. Everybody can ask the Federal Ministry for Consumer Protection, the Federal Ministry for Health, etc., for scientific evidence that justifies the bird flu panic.

If you wait for "others" to do something, you shouldn't be surprised if the others don't do anything and the situation not only doesn't stay the way it is now, but is also getting much worse. Ultimately, we as citizens are behind this, because we have been watching all this insanity happening around us for years without doing anything. We have to start taking social responsibility if we don't want to surrender to and be the victims of the total dominance and the chaos of an uncontrolled pseudoscience.

194

Considering this, *do you think we have to fight science?*

The dominance of the pseudoscience has to be overcome by a social science that is determined by its commitment to be honest, checkable, and traceable.

The language of the present traditional medicine reveals its focus on the democratic-constitutional uncontrolled dominance when traditional physicians and the state refer to the *"dominant opinion in medical science"* we have to submit to, and when this dominance claims that the stork brings the babies, or that earth is flat.

But we don't have any reason to complain. After all, we tolerate this behaviour of the state. However, if people continue to tolerate that we are to surrender to this dominance like we currently do in the absurd case of the bird flu claims, nobody should be surprised to wake up one morning, horrified at the realization that he or she is dead: Killed by the dominance he or she as a citizen of a democratic constitutional state tolerated.

In a democratic constitutional state, the bird flu panic would be just as impossible as AIDS and vaccinations. We as citizens have to put the constitutional state into effect. Only then, neither AIDS, nor the pseudoscience and the bird flu have a chance. The only thing I can say is: Don't give bird flu a chance! Don't believe the lies they tell you! Check it! Use your brain!

For those who want to do something: You can find suggestions at: www.agenda-leben.de.

© 2005 FAKTuell ® Die Onlinezeitung

195

In Preparation for Publication:

factor-L – The New Medicine
The Truth about Dr. Hamer's Discovery
Cancer and other curable diseases
Monika Berger-Lenz * Christopher Ray * Prof. Dr. H. U. Niemitz

It needs a little bit of luck to come across Dr. Ryke Geerd Hamer's New Medicine. Of course, a certain amount of curiosity and access to the Internet is also necessary - the latter is not to be underestimated! For, neither the TV nor the radio, neither magazines nor periodicals, neither newspapers nor professional journals offer information about this discovery. And although some people would like to dismiss it as being quackery, most prefer to keep quiet about it rather than openly demonize it. That isn't really surprising considering the consequences of this discovery by the ingenious doctor from Frisia. Dr. Ryke Geerd Hamer gave humankind a gift that has been withheld from people to date. But nobody has to accept that; the personal stories in this book prove it.

Doctors and practitioners of alternative medicine gave us the opportunity to get in contact with those of their patients who use Dr. Hamer's New Medicine.

The result: 18 people told their stories. They are not all about cancer; they are also about allergies or learning difficulties, just to mention a few. The stories show that the biological laws of the New Medicine apply in every case. For people who concern themselves with the natural laws and understand them, earth won't be flat any longer from now on.

With an introduction to the New Medicine and Professor Dr. Hans-Ulrich Niemitz's scientific expert opinion regarding the New Medicine.

Table of Contents

Conflicts and Solutions - In Practice

FAKTuell-Verlag
We make it easy!

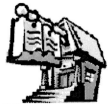

FAKTuell ® Verlag
Monika Berger-Lenz
An den Birken 5
D-02827 Görlitz
Germany

Phone: +49 3581-40 22 40
Fax: +49 3581-40 22 42

***

Internet:
FAKTuell.de
faktor-L.de
ketario.de
faktuell-verlag.de

***

E-Mail:
CvD@ FAKTuell.de

***

ISBN: 978-3-9809203-3-9
(2006: ISBN: 3-9809203-3-X)
EAN: 9783980920399
©2005 by FAKTuell
All rights reserved

***

FAKTuell ® is a registered trademark of the FAKTuell editorial department Berger-Lenz

Lightning Source UK Ltd.
Milton Keynes UK
UKOW02f1833300115

245438UK00001B/118/P